Vaginal Surgery

Vaginal Surgery

Michel Cosson
Gynecological Surgeon
Jeanne-de-Flandre Hospital, Lille, France

Denis Querleu
Gynecological Surgeon,
Cancer Center of the Claudius-Regaud Institute, Toulouse, France

Daniel Dargent
Formerly Director of Gynecology and Obstetrics
Edouard-Herriot Hospital, Lyon, France

Illustrations by Guillaume Blanchet

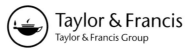

Taylor & Francis
Taylor & Francis Group

Boca Raton London New York Singapore

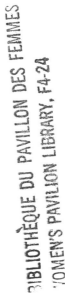

This is a English translation of a book originally published in French, titled, Chirurgie Vaginale, authored by M. Cosson, D. Querleu, and D. Dargent, published by Masson, 2003, Issy-Les Maoulineaux, France

Published in 2005 by
Taylor & Francis Group
6000 Broken Sound Parkway NW, Suite 300
Boca Raton, FL 33487-2742

International Standard Book Number-10: 0-8247-1984-0 (Hardcover)
International Standard Book Number-13: 978-0-8247-1984-5 (Hardcover)

Library of Congress Cataloging-in-Publication Data

Catalog record is available from the Library of Congress

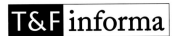

Visit the Taylor & Francis Web site at
http://www.taylorandfrancis.com

Taylor & Francis Group is the Academic Division of T&F Informa plc.

Preface

To compose the preface of a work represents, for the person who is so honored, an exercise that is at once uplifting, dangerous and uncertain. Uplifting, because it gives the pleasurable but ephemeral impression of possessing an immense power of judgment. Dangerous, because he must summarize, with great economy, the main points of the elements of the matter without allowing his personal emotions to interfere. And uncertain because the one and real judge of the work will always be the reader himself.

For the specific case of the subject of vaginal surgery, the task has been greatly facilitated by the level of excellence of the criteria of judgment. The subject: to have selected, the theme of gynecological surgery via vaginal access for a book with a pedagogical vocation has proven to be an excellent opportunity. In fact, gynecological surgery, after a long period of domination by the "abdominal approach" has benefited from two major aspects of its evolution:

1. The appearance of laparoscopy. This technique has radically changed a certain number of therapeutic procedures and has now found its place, precisely targeted but not exclusive.

2. The renaissance in France of vaginal surgery. Developed for many years in the Germanic countries, it has found its footing in France largely thanks to Daniel Dargent who, with his characteristic spirit of tenacity, successfully convinced a number of French surgical teams to adopt these techniques.

The subject is treated, not as a partisan argument but rather as an update of all the possibilities available to this route of non-scarring surgical access, without, at the same time, refusing to recognize the role of recourse or partnership that laparoscopic techniques can play.

The authors, Michel Cosson, Denis Querleu, Daniel Dargent, provide, with the strength of their credentials, a development of their experiences, their ideas, their convictions, and above all they demonstrate impressive objectivity that brings an appropriate perspective to tried and tested techniques. In addition, the authors have avoided the classic trap of wanting to present the very latest trends and instead focus with critical judgment on known and validated procedures, and not to place too much emphasis on innovative solutions that become somewhat widespread even before their validity has been properly shown.

The editorial preparation of this work has been impeccable by its quality and the precision of its illustrations and documentation, but also for its concern to keep "glued" together the text with the act in order to facilitate the imaginative recreation of the surgical technique within a static document.

With the points that they share in common, it is not surprising that these three names have been united under the authorship of this single book and this in despite of appearances. First of all, I count all three as friends, and two as former students, to find them together as accomplices for such an endeavor offers me both feelings of joy and inexpressible pride. They are, all three, passionate about surgery and more generally about the profession of a surgeon, rigorous in their approach, honest with themselves about their results, and perfectly convincing in their argumentation and demonstration. They have a common, permanent concern for the transmission to younger generations of their knowledge and know-how by stressing the quality of communication and conviviality. This work on surgery should be received as a manual and a constant companion, one of the most authentic methods of the teaching of medicine. All of the procedures discussed herein have the great advantage of being reproducible—even if a certain number of the operations (the Watkins, for example) are practiced by a relatively small number of practitioners—and thus earning the label of "sound surgical practice."

The authors have benefited from a solid gynaecology/obstetrics education, providing them with the profound knowledge and experience needed to relate to the aspirations, worries and hopes of women as they come to face their gynecologic life, especially when pathologies are concerned. This irreplaceable experience provides them with the astuteness required to make wise and qualified surgical decisions.

One of the authors, in spite of his immense surgical talent, accepts the role as "regional gynaecologist": apart from being a grand act of modesty, this is a wonderful tribute to the specialisation and, more simply, to women in general, regardless of what their expectations might be.

Thus, by the collaboration of three talented players, this work represents the realisation of a dream that would have been inaccessible to a single author while still fully immersed in a surgical career. To all those practising or wishing to practise gynaecological surgery, it offers a global and human vision and an approach to woman's surgery, without succumbing to the temptation of sub-dividing the field into rival specialisations. Furthermore, it is an ardent plea for an approach to surgery where the patient is more important than the surgical intervention. Finally, it is a most precious contribution to modern gynaecological surgery and to the spirit that will safeguard the medicine of tomorrow.

Professor Gilles Crépin

Table of Contents

Preface, Gilles Crépin

Surgical environment

PART 1

CHAPTER 1

Immediate pre- and postoperative care

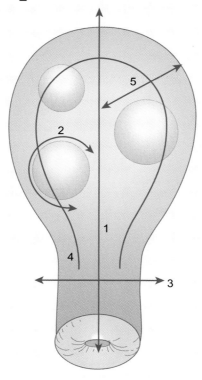

1.1 *Techniques used for reducing uterine volume.*
1. Hemisection.   2. Myomectomy.   3. Cervical amputation.   4. Endometrial Coring.   5. Uterine morcellation.

Guide for the reader

1. This chapter presents the basis required for the preparatory stages of a procedure.
2. Even if a vaginal operation is usually itself benign in the case of a benign pathology, it presents certain risks that must be anticipated – in particular infection (contamination of surgical origin) and thromboembolism.

The first, preparative stage of a surgical procedure is above all psychological, with information provided about the indications and long-term consequences of the surgical procedure. In the presence of anaemia caused by genital haemorrhage, a preliminary treatment to induce amenorrhea could be an effective means of preventing transfusions, as long as there is no therapeutic emergency connected to a malignant pathology. The preparatory prescription of estrogens before surgery of the prolapse forms part of certain protocols, applied in order to improve the trophicity and scarring of the tissue.

PREPARATION

A shower shortly before the operation, the pre-operative antiseptic cleansing of the vagina, and the strict adherence to antiseptic procedures in general form part of the effort to prevent infection. An antibiotic that acts on Gram-negative and anaerobic germs needs to be applied. However, post-operative antibiotic therapy is not justified, even in the presence of a vesical catheter.

ANAESTHESIA

The operation can be performed equally well under general or loco-regional anaesthesia; indeed, vaginal surgery is particularly well suited for application of spinal anaesthesia (provided that the duration of the intervention does not exceed two hours) or epidural anaesthesia. However, tensions on the ovarian pedicles and intraperitoneal manipulations can be painful if the anaesthesia is insufficient. Although surveillance is part of standard procedure, special care will be taken during periods of variable venous flow, namely during the positioning and re-positioning of the inferior limbs.

PAIN

The period following an operation can be painful, even after simple vaginal hysterectomy and, *a fortiori*, after complex treatment of a prolapse, including intense perineal pain that is sometimes aggravated by hemorrhoidal growth. Nothing can prevent such pain, if only efficient teamwork that includes anaesthesiologists. Broad prescription of strong analgesic

drugs, or, if necessary, of self-administrable intravenous (PCA) or epidural (PCEA) drugs, must already be envisaged during the anaesthetics consultation. The psychological effects, the positioning on the operating table, the strong tensions, the extensive separations, and closing sutures represent risk factors for the occurrence of postoperative pains that have to be taken into account, even though this is a minimally invasive operation.

POSTOPERATIVE SURVEILLANCE

Included as a part of the postoperative surveillance are the intestinal functions, abdominal state, urinary function, and arterial blood pressure, as well as the body temperature. Postoperative vaginal discharge is more or less bloody and can last for several weeks, but is of little concern. Urinary retention is frequent following treatment of a prolapse, rare but possible following simple complete hysterectomy, and there is no need to place an indwelling catheter: only 10% of the patients will have to be catheterized during the evening after the procedure, and more often than not, catheterisation will not be required again thereafter. Following the treatment of a prolapse or radical hysterectomy, it is recommended to place an indwelling catheter for 48 hours. After its removal, micturition will be closely monitored in order to avoid any hyperextension of the bladder wall. Post-micturational residues must be measured until below 100 ml two times consecutively or below 50 ml. In case of urinary retention, self-catheterisation must be taught. Of course, this is only possible with patients where general health, psychological state and coordination indicate high chances for the successful learning of self-catheterisation methods. This also helps the patient to view the urinary retention with less anguish and aids with rapid recovery.

Rising and release from hospitalisation

Early rising and early food intake, as well as the prophylaxis of thromboembolic accidents are standard. The duration of postoperative hospitalisation is variable. Certain groups on the American continents have practiced simple complete hysterectomy on an outpatient basis. Such an extreme situation can only be applied under favourable social situations, for example in cases where home care is provided and where the general conditions and accommodation at home are appropriate; although it is possible to leave the hospital on the first day, the patient is most frequently discharged between the second and fourth day following the procedure. Radical hysterectomy also allows for short hospitalisation, the only constraint being the necessity of self-catheterisation in the case of urinary retention. Following treatment of a prolapse, hospitalisation is longer due to age, pain, urinary retention and greater difficulties of mobility.

CHAPTER 2

Positioning

Guide for the reader

Abdominal surgery is carried out on a structure that is flat overall: a surface is delimited by four exclusion sheets; since the patient, when lying flat, provides an almost ideally planar surface, the view is direct and without obstacle, so that the surgeon and assistant surgeon can easily place themselves on either side for optimal access. An analogous result should be obtained for vaginal surgery by correct positioning of the patient. The secret lies in eliminating the obstacle created by the inferior limbs.

Depending on the surgeon's preference and size, he may either sit or stand. The assisting surgeons must also be taken into account when choosing the surgeon's position: they will have to bend over if the surgeon is both short and sitting, whereas if he is tall and standing, they will need to stand, stretching on tiptoe in order to provide appropriate assistance. The height of the operating table is adjusted accordingly, approximately at the height of the surgeon's elbows. If possible, two assistant surgeons should be present, with one on either side of the surgeon, as well as an instrument nurse positioned behind the surgeon's right or left shoulder, depending on whether he is right- or left-handed. The instrument nurse is provided with a table that is placed behind the surgeon's back. A good instrument nurse will know the procedure from start to finish and prepare the instruments and sutures in anticipation of the surgeon's requests. The advantage of such an ideal set-up is that the surgeon can fully concentrate on an operating field that remains constantly in his view.

POSITIONING OF THE PATIENT

Correct positioning of the patient is a fundamental concern. The patient is placed in *dorsal decubitus*, with the buttocks protruding over the edge of the operating table. The classical gynaecological position would suffice for providing the surgeon with a good view, but the position of the patient's inferior limbs would completely hamper efficient assistance by the assistant surgeons. This is noteworthy because the assistant surgeons are of major importance during vaginal surgery (two assistant surgeons are required for every major operation). Therefore, the patient must be positioned with the inferior limbs removed as far as possible from the operation field so as not to impede the assistant surgeons. The two possible positions are as follows:

– in the first, the thighs are angled at 90°, the legs positioned vertically, the feet suspended by stirrups;
– in the second, more relevant to the characteristics of modern tables, *gynecological leg supports* are used. The flexion at the thigh is increased, with slight abduction, leaving the legs resting on the supports in a slightly bent position. The inferior limbs are maintained above the vertical plane defined by the operating table's edge (*figure 2.1*).

An antiseptic solution is applied from the suprapubic region to the furrow between the buttocks, and laterally across the internal

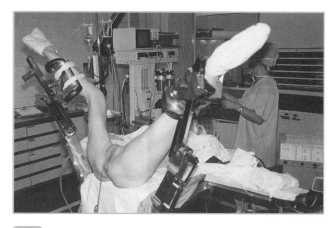

2.1 Positioning on the gynecological leg supports.

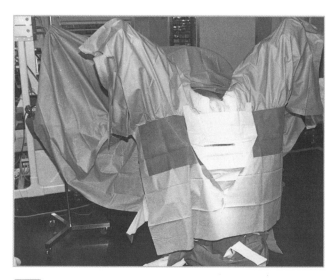

2.2 The same position, after placement of the exclusion sheets.

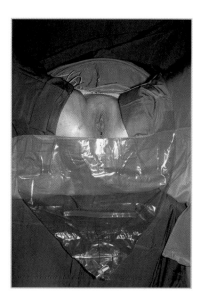

2.3 Close-up view of the operating field.

surfaces of the thighs. The exclusion sheets must be adapted to vaginal surgery: one is placed under the buttocks to ensure a tight seal between the patient and the table, the inferior limbs are completely covered, and another sheet covers the abdomen (*figure 2.2*). A collecting pouch allows one to measure blood loss and to prevent the loss of instruments (*figure 2.3*).

The assistant surgeons (*figure 2.4*) must be able to view and stand in a natural, untwisted position next to the surgeon. The table's height, the surgeon's decision to sit or stand, as well as the placement of the patient's legs, are all important factors in this consideration.

PRECAUTIONS

One must, in all cases, prevent the compression of nerves and the dangerous syndrome related to poorly adjusted leg supports, which should not be too firmly adjusted or left under direct pressure at the contact points. This falls under the responsibility of the surgeon, who must inform the nurses and prepare a precise procedure involving the use of foams and gels as necessary. Patients suffering from sciatic pain must be identified preoperatively and informed of the risk for at least transitorily elevated pains: in such cases, straining positions must be avoided, while maintaining the surgeon's visual field. The thin loops can be removed by placing the patient in a modified Trendelenburg position, thus bringing the vaginal axis into the axis of the lighting. The use of a suction cannula is advisable: the operational field during vaginal surgery is narrow and therefore easily obscured; compresses would only be in the way and obstruct access.

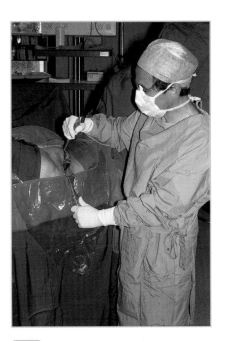

2.4 Position of the assistant surgeons.

CHAPTER 3

Instrumentation

Guide for the reader

Vaginal surgery without the specific instruments would be like laparoscopic surgery without the specific forceps and scissors. Use of badly adapted retractors can result in serious difficulty and even prove dangerous.

Vaginal surgery does not require many specialised instruments, since all fixation and clamp forceps, needle-holders and scissors are part of the standard equipment. However, some instruments are indispensable, in particular the retractors.

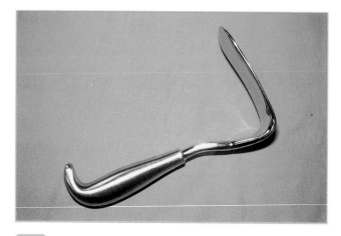

3.1 "Posterior" Mangiagalli retractor.

THE RETRACTORS, ESSENTIAL INSTRUMENTS

Contrary to laparotomy, the general principle of vaginal surgery allows the viewing of only a minor part of the operating field at a time, namely the one being treated. The sector of interest is revealed with the help of retractors, which explains their absolute necessity. Retractors are required for two applications during vaginal surgery. One retractor must be placed in the Douglas' pouch where it should maintain its position on its own without being in the way: the ideal retractor for this purpose is the Mangiagalli retractor, which is bent at a 45° angle (*Figure 3.1*). All other retractors must flatten away the vaginal walls and viscera, all the while making sure that the assistant surgeons' hands do not the hamper access to the operating field. Therefore, bayonet-shaped retractors, such as the Breisky retractors, are the ideal choice. They come in different sizes, concerning both the blade's width and length, which are especially adapted for successive surgical steps (*Figures 3.2 and 3.3*). The minimum requirements are two retractors measuring 28 x 80 mm and one measuring 32 x 90 mm. The following retractors are also useful: very thin (15 mm) and very broad (40 mm).

DECHAMP'S NEEDLE

Since vaginal surgery is sometimes quite deep, Dechamp's Neddles are used, the most common of which is the Deschamps needle with large curvature. Similar to forceps, it is held between two fingers, and its padded tip prevents damage to the tissues it penetrates (*Figure 3.4*).

Beware of imitations of this instrument, since its perfect efficiency depends on the precision of its wide curvature, allowing for a considerable range of angle. A lateral shift is allowable, but the curvature in the plane of the grip is satisfactory and versatile.

FORCEPS

Tension forceps are useful for the manipulation of the edges of the incision during removal of a prolapse or during cancer surgery (*Figure 3.5*). Allis forceps or long Kocher forceps are

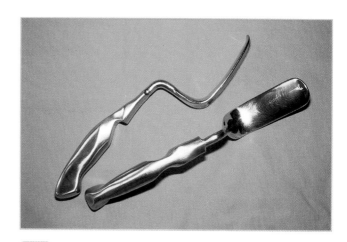

3.2 Breisky retractor.

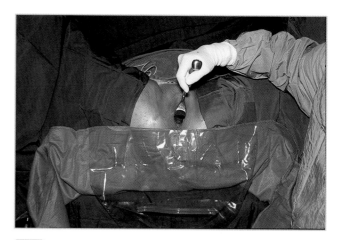

3.3 Correct handling of a Breisky retractor.

ideal instruments for this purpose, at the same time offering efficiency and reducing traumatism; four such forceps are required. For radical vaginal hysterectomy, forceps with large, strong teeth are indispensable for drawing close and isolating the vaginal neck: a set of six Chroback forceps is useful. Since access to the uterine wall or to myomas can prove difficult, a set of Pozzi forceps and Museux forceps should be available.

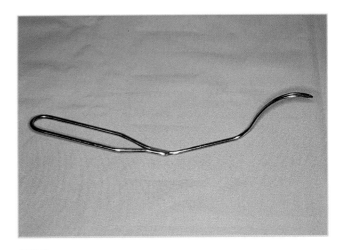

3.4   The vaginal Deschamps needle.

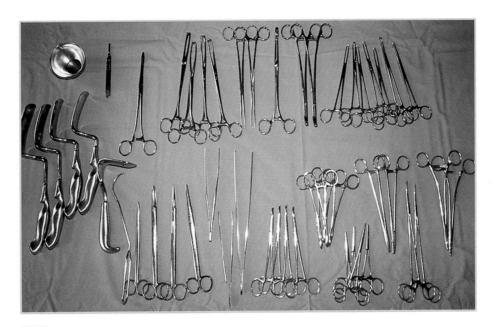

3.5   The complete set of instruments.

CHAPTER 4

Specific anatomy and the creation of spaces

Guide for the reader

The special features of the vaginal surgery are twofold.

1. The anatomy is viewed upside down (from bottom to top) as compared to standard textbook descriptions (from top to bottom); it is, therefore, necessary to learn to conceptually visualize the anatomy as a "mirror image".

2. Access to pelvic organs is thus different: while for abdominal surgery the abdomen is opened by incision, one has to rethink access routes during vaginal surgery. "Vaginal" surgery is actually not the appropriate term: one either works through the vaginal canal, thus performing *transvaginal surgery*, or through the pelvic floor, thus performing *perineal surgery*.

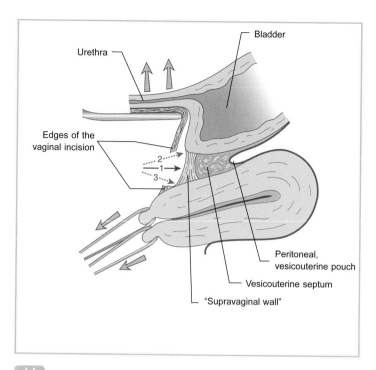

Urethra

Bladder

Edges of the
vaginal incision

2
1
3

Peritoneal,
vesicouterine pouch

Vesicouterine septum

"Supravaginal wall"

4.1 The "supravaginal wall".
The opposing pulls of the uterine cervix (downwards) and the edge of the vaginal incision (upwards) reveals connective tissue, namely the supravaginal wall, which must be penetrated in order to reach the vesicouterine septum. This obstacle will be removed by sectioning the fibers in the median plane, half-way between the uterus and the vaginal pouch (arrow 1). Should this rule not be followed, the incision passes incorrectly either to the bladder (arrow 2) or the uterus (arrow 3).
1. Correct direction.
2. Wrong direction.
3. Wrong direction.

SPECIFIC ANATOMY

Apart from the different approach conditions and angles of view, the anatomy of vaginal surgery is the same as that of conventional abdominal surgery: one will thus encounter the paravisceral fossae of Latzko, as well as the septa that are familiar to abdominal surgeons. The one basic difference is the effect of the tensions exerted on the uterine cervix, based on its connection to the bladder, as well as on the position of the ureter. Bladder injuries are relatively frequent in vaginal surgery, while damage to the ureter is relatively rare: adequate knowledge of the anatomy will prevent both.

The bladder

Tension on the uterine cervix lowers the bladder's floor and results in a thickening of the vesicouterine septum (by condensation of the connective tissue), which creates a transversal pseudo-ligament called the supracervical or supravaginal wall (figures 4.1 and 4.2). This pseudo-ligament is made more prominent by placing a retractor below the urethra (figure 4.1) and using forceps to grasp the edge of the vaginal incision on the median line in order to firmly pull it upwards. This displaces the bladder, forming a bulge that is at risk of rupture (figure 4.1). This bulge can be pushed back by sectioning the supravaginal septum fibres from the cervix and uterine isthmus. The thus defined supravaginal septum is very limited in height (about one centimeter) when approached directly from the cervico-vaginal junction, as is the case during hysterectomy without colpectomy. If the vagina is incised further down, the supracervical wall appears longer and the risk of vesical injury proportionately greater.

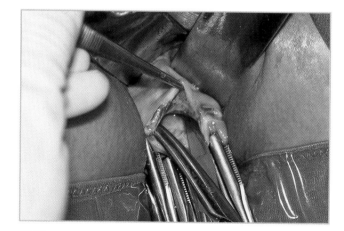

4.2 The "supravaginal wall".
The downward pull of the uterine cervix, the pressure of the anterior retractor on the bladder, and the grasp of dissection forceps on the central part of the edge of the vaginal incision provide the three key points of identification of the supravaginal wall.

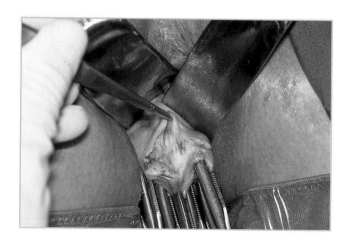

4.3 Access to the vesicouterine septum.
Following a complete median section of the supravaginal wall, a retractor can be placed in the vesicouterine septum. The peritoneal pouch is located at the end of this septum.

Complete section of the "supravaginal wall" reveals the vesicouterine septum and, higher up, the peritoneal vesicouterine pouch (*figure 4.3*). The vesicouterine septum communicates laterally with the broad ligament (*figures 4.4 and 4.5*). Access to the vesicouterine septum thus represents one of the key techniques in vaginal surgery: if successful, it provides a good median view onto the uterine isthmus as well as a lateral view onto the uterine pedicle; if unsuccessful, it will be haemorrhagic and dangerous to both the bladder and ureter.

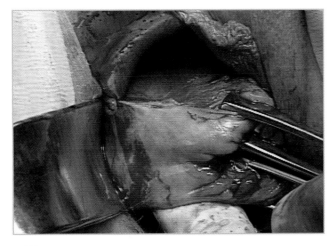

4.4 Vesicouterine septum, access to the broad ligament.
This is the key representation of vaginal surgery and will be shown repeatedly in different chapters. The vesicouterine septum is open and a retractor has been placed therein. The bladder is thus protected. In order to reach the pars flaccida of the broad ligament, one merely needs to tilt this retractor sideways.

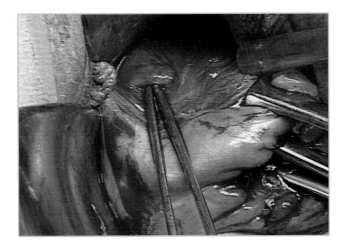

4.5 Vesicouterine septum, access to the broad ligament.
Pushing the bladder pillar (vesicouterine ligament) laterally, together with the ureter contained therein, the contents of broad ligament are visualised, and in particular the loop of the uterine artery.

The ureter

The ureter is the potential victim of hysterectomies and serves as a reference point for paracervical ablation during cancer surgery. Transposition of the general anatomical concepts concerning the pelvic tissue and the terminal ureter are required during a vaginal approach. The difference lies in the fact that, during an abdominal approach, the ureter is located under the descending part of the uterine artery, pulled upwards by the tensions. Thus, the ureter "descends" regularly from the edge of the pelvis until it reaches its terminal segment – its lowest point – where is shows a practically horizontal orientation.

During a vaginal approach, the ureter is located between the surgeon and the uterine artery, which is pulled downwards by the tensions, while the bladder is pushed upwards by the retractors. The connective fibres that accompany the uterine artery and the vesicouterine ligament (which inserts itself onto the bladder near the ureter's ending) cause the formation of a ureteral loop known by the surgical name "ureteral knee" (*figure 4.6*). The lowest point is thus located about 2 to 3 cm from the ureter's end point. Since the tensions' effect remains small, the loop is rather wide and the "knee" is 1 to 2 cm below the ureteral ending. The anatomy can thus be summarised as follows: the ureter descends along the dorso-lateral side of the pelvis, forms its loop under the uterine artery, and ascends again towards the ventral part where it joins the bladder. The

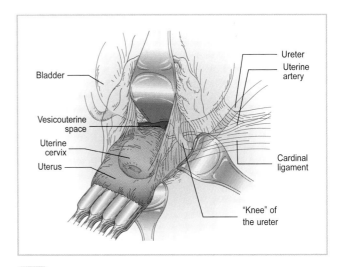

Bladder

Vesicouterine space

Uterine cervix

Uterus

Ureter

Uterine artery

Cardinal ligament

"Knee" of the ureter

4.6 The bladder pillar and its contents.

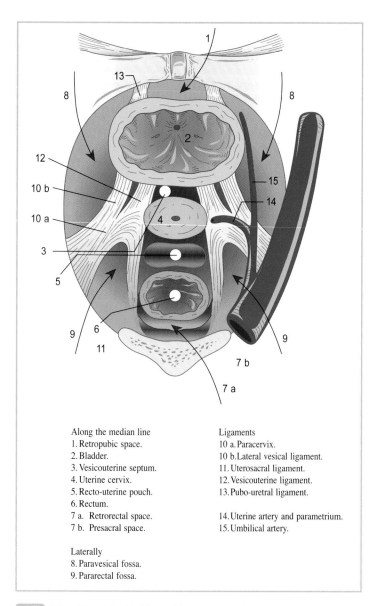

Along the median line
1. Retropubic space.
2. Bladder.
3. Vesicouterine septum.
4. Uterine cervix.
5. Recto-uterine pouch.
6. Rectum.
7 a. Retrorectal space.
7 b. Presacral space.

Laterally
8. Paravesical fossa.
9. Pararectal fossa.

Ligaments
10 a. Paracervix.
10 b. Lateral vesical ligament.
11. Uterosacral ligament.
12. Vesicouterine ligament.
13. Pubo-uretral ligament.

14. Uterine artery and parametrium.
15. Umbilical artery.

4.7 The pillar of the bladder and its contents. Pelvic spaces and ligaments

pushed towards the right of the vesico-vaginal septum, and the left ureter when pushed towards the left *(figure 4.4)*; this motion can be performed with precision and efficiency only when the peritoneal pouch remains intact: it should, therefore, not be incised during the preparation for hysterectomy;

– the uterine artery is accessed at the level of its loop, halfway between the ureter and the lateral side of the isthmus.

By following these two rules, traumatism to ureters occurs only rarely during non-radical vaginal surgery.

SPACES, SEPTA, FASCIAS, LIGAMENTS

Whichever the approach, the surgeon is presented with two types of pelvic cellular tissue: soft regions, which can be exploited to progress into the depths of the surgical field, and dense regions (fascias and visceral "ligaments"), which either need to be cut during dissection or ablation, or can be used for reparative surgery.

Six parietal spaces (two median, four lateral), as well as two intervisceral spaces or septa are considered *(figure 4.7)*:

– the retropubic space (Retzius' space), located behind the pubic symphysis and in front of the bladder; famous for its dangerous veins, it is actually nearly completely avascular, since the vesical veins are in contact with the bladder and urethra.

– the two paravesical fossae, whose superior orifice (as seen during abdominal surgery) is located between the umbilical artery on the inside and the iliac vascular axis on the outside. They are large and deep, with the levator ani muscle and its aponeurosis forming their floor, and they are crossed by the vasculo-nervous obturator pedicle.

– the two pararectal fossae, which have a narrow abdominal orifice, are located in the sacro-iliac sinus, between the wall and vessels laterally and the rectum medially; the sacrum provides their dorsal wall, while their floor is formed by the sacro-coccygeal insertion of the pelvic floor; during vaginal surgery one has access to their caudal part, which is broader outside the vagina, above the plane of the levators; the central rectal pedicle, which marks the lateral rectal ligament, is situated at the junction between the upper and lower parts.

– the retrorectal space is located between the rectal fascia and the retrorectal fascia; disrupting it all the way to the ano-coccygeal raphe does not present any risk; further dorsally, between the retrorectal fascia and the sacrum, lies the presacral space which is dangerous due to the presence of the sacral veins;

– the vesicovaginal and vesicouterine septum (or space) is located under the median part of the anterior peritoneal

uterine artery, coming from the pelvic wall, appears to "emerge from" the loop.

During simple hysterectomy, the terminal ureter is protected in two ways:

– the sectioning of the supravaginal wall results in the mobilizing of the bladder's floor, allowing a retractor to be placed under the fornix in the vesicouterine septum. This retractor lifts and, more importantly, laterally displaces the right ureter when

pouch, behind the vesical floor; at the bottom it is delimited by the tight connection between urethra and vagina;
– the rectovaginal septum or space is located between the upper two thirds of the vagina and the rectum; the joining of the uterosacral ligaments behind the uterine cervix limits its access during an abdominal approach, while adhesion of the vagina to the anal canal above the perineum's tendinous centre limits its access during a vaginal approach.

Zones of areolar connective tissue are not spaces in an anatomical sense. They are normally filled with soft tissue that represents a flexible intervisceral and vesico-parietal link, providing the basis of the pelvic statics or, rather, its dynamics. The surgeon will create "spaces" or "pouches" by opening these zones of areolar connective tissue using the tip of scissors, of forceps, or of his fingers. Mastering their access is one of the key steps in pelvic surgery. To summarise what is to be detailed below, several opening techniques must be mastered:
– from a vaginal approach, access to the pouches is easiest along the paracervix: immediately at its ventral side for the paravesical fossa, and at its dorsal side for the pararectal fossa;
– this access is located exactly at the vagina's deep surface; it is bloodless: any wrong path taken when moving away from the vagina is marked by bleeding;
– a correct opening in the right direction is always extremely easy: the pouch appears to "swallow" the scissors; necessity for physical effort of any kind indicates a wrong path;
– there is one (and only one) difference in anatomical arrangement between the abdominal and vaginal approaches: the paravesical fossa has a wide abdominal and a narrow vaginal orifice, while the pararectal fossa exhibits a narrow abdominal and a wide vaginal orifice.

Fascias

The fascias are the connective layers enveloping viscera and muscles. The term includes the viscera's adventitia and the muscles' epimysium, the term aponeurosis being, anatomically speaking, strictly reserved for the fibrous muscular insertions. The visceral fascias (rectal, vaginal, uterine, urethral, and vesical) and fascias of the pelvic diaphragm (previously called "pelvic aponeurosis") are known as the pelvic fascias. They are of variable thickness and distorted in cases of genito-pelvic prolapse, especially along the median line. Visceral and pelvic fascias exchange fibres in several zones, which are both narrow anatomic connections – requiring surgical dissection and representing a risk of visceral rupture – and dynamic connections between the pelvic diaphragm and the viscera:

– at the points where each viscera crosses the pelvic fascia;
– between vagina and urethra and vesical neck;
– between vagina and anal canal.

Figure 4.8 shows the limits of the subperitoneal pelvic space: the pelvic diaphragm and its fascia at the bottom, the pelvic peritoneum at the top. One can thus visualise why a peritoneal incision suffices to provide access to the subperitoneal pelvic space during an abdominal approach, while during a vaginal approach one needs to disrupt the endopelvic fascia's parietal insertion in the periphery.

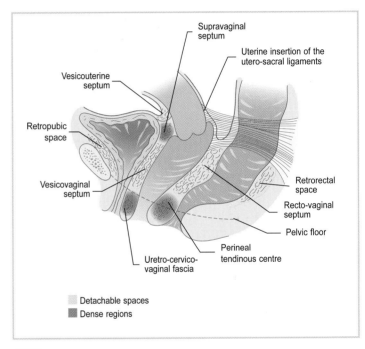

Supravaginal septum

Uterine insertion of the utero-sacral ligaments

Vesicouterine septum

Retropubic space

Vesicovaginal septum

Retrorectal space

Recto-vaginal septum

Pelvic floor

Uretro-cervico-vaginal fascia

Perineal tendinous centre

◻ Detachable spaces
◼ Dense regions

4.8 Boundaries of the subperitoneal pelvic space. Median sagittal section of the pelvis.

Ligaments

The visceral "ligaments" are connective reinforcements of the pelvic cellular tissue: they are, therefore, continuous with the areolar tissue and, above all, with the fascias.

Thus, the pelvic ligaments are not articulate ligaments, but rather represent dense connective zones whose visceral insertion joins the perivisceral fascia, and whose parietal insertion is often negligible. They may be modified by the course of pathology, and application of tension during surgery results in their separation, reinforcing the surgeon's impression to be dealing with a "ligament". The pelvic cellular tissue resembles a mesh network: the meshes approach when pulling at one point, resulting in densification of the structure.

All these ligaments exchange fibres between each other as well as with the fascias. Their boundaries are, therefore, not precisely definable. The best characterised example is the

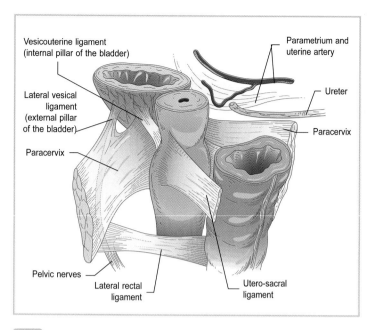

Vesicouterine ligament
(internal pillar of the bladder)

Lateral vesical
ligament
(external pillar
of the bladder)

Paracervix

Pelvic nerves

Lateral rectal
ligament

Parametrium and
uterine artery

Ureter

Paracervix

Utero-sacral
ligament

4.9 "Ligamentous" structures of the pelvis.

The visceral ligaments can be divided into two groups: the lateral ligaments, accompanied by the internal iliac terminal arteries, and the sagittal ligaments that carry the nerves of the hypogastric plexus (*figures 4.7 and 4.9*).

In theory, there are three lateral ligaments: rectal, genital and vesical.

The genital ligament is the most complex. It consists of three aligned parts: the parametrium accompanies the uterine artery, the lower paracervix ("cardinal ligament", "Mackenrodt ligament", also referred to as "parametrium" by surgeons) consists of a dense cervical segment and a thinner vaginal segment, the latter of which is often referred to as "paracolpos" or paravagina. This ligament is not strictly transversal, but , similar to the branching of the hypogastric artery, originates from the dorso-lateral wall of the pelvis. In fact, it is not really a "ligament" in the articular sense. It consists of pelvic visceral vessels and node-bearing fatty tissue, and it contains pelvic autonomic nerves.

The vesical ligament appears to be inserted onto the parametrium, that it leaves in a forward direction together with the umbilico-vesical artery, half-way between the wall and the uterus, outside of the ureter; it forms the external column of the bladder, also known as the "anterior parametrium".

The rectal ligament is inserted further down in the sacroiliac sinus and, together with the median rectal artery and rectal nerves, constitutes the wing of the rectum. The sagittal ligaments are formed by the utero-sacral and vesicouterine ligaments. Together with a hypothetical pubovesical ligament, this complex is called the "sacropubic lamina", even though it is neither a lamina, nor sacro-, nor pubic... The uterosacral ligaments contain connective tissue and the nerves of the lower hypogastric plexus, but only few blood vessels. Sometimes, they weakly insert themselves in a fan-like fashion into the sacral holes S2 through S4, bypassing the rectum by exchanging fibres with the rectal fascia and the lateral rectal ligament, and running along the recto-uterine pouch (Douglas' pouch) before inserting themselves into the vaginal pouch close to the median line of the isthmus by exchange of fibres with the pericervical fascia and the paracervix. The vesicouterine ligaments attach the lateral sides of the isthmus and uterine cervix to the region of the ureteral meatus. They form the internal columns of the bladder.

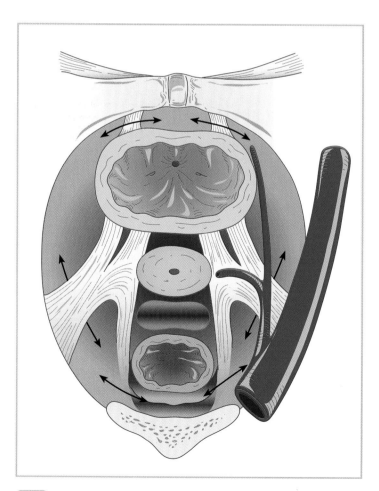

4.10 Communication between spaces.

uterine cervix's connective apparatus: the pericervical and perivaginal fascia is the direct extension of the utero-sacral ligaments and the two paracervices, and it exchanges fibres with the pelvic fascia. This explains why ablation of the uterine cervix does not result in a prolapse: the fascias that keep the remaining vaginal vault in suspension are not disturbed.

Communication between spaces

The architectural organisation of these different structures provides portals of entry and of communication between spaces (figures 4.10 and 4.11).

The communication between the vesicouterine septum and the broad ligament has already been discussed (cf. figure 4.4).

The paracervix separates the paravesical fossa from the pararectal pouch. Being arranged in an oblique fashion, the paravesical fossa presents a wide and the pararectal fossa a narrow opening to the abdominal surgeon (the opposite is true during a vaginal approach). Towards the lower end, the separation is not absolute: between the paracervix and the pelvic diaphragm lies a passage connecting the two fossa. The parietal spaces are connected to each other as follows: either side of the paravesical fossae with the retropubic space; the paravesical fossae with the pararectal fossae below the paracervices; and the pararectal fossae with the retrorectal space.

The utero-sacral ligaments only partially separate the pararectal fossae from the retrorectal and presacral spaces. In fact, these spaces communicate nearly without interruption. The apparent insertion of these ligaments is in fact made up of autonomic nerves, which can be protected by keeping them against the pelvic wall and approaching the rectum exactly at the border of the mesorectum; this is a key technique of rectal cancer surgery.

Pelvic diaphragm

Seen from below, the pelvic diaphragm (figure 4.12) reveals mainly its internal levator and the pubic insertions. The pubo-vaginal and puborectal muscles surround the urogenital cleft. The visceral fascias are directly accessible by incision through the vaginal wall, whose adventice is itself a fascia. In front, the fascias are laterally inserted into the ischiopubic rami. In the ventro-lateral plane, one needs to disrupt the visceral fascias in order to reach the levator muscle's pubic insertion, and to disrupt the pelvic fascias to reach the Retzius space and para-vesical pouches.

In the dorso-lateral plane, the levator is located much lower, since its direction in a woman in an upright position is nearly vertical; the vaginal lower third is opposite the pelvic diaphragm, while the two upper thirds are opposite the pararectal fossae. The latter is defined medially by the rectum, towards the head by the paracervix, and laterally by the pelvic wall (more specifically the ischio-coccygeal muscle containing the sacrospinal ligament). The best approach to attain this ligament is, therefore, via the pararectal fossa.

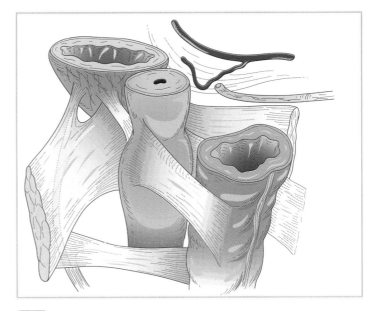

4.11 Communication between spaces.

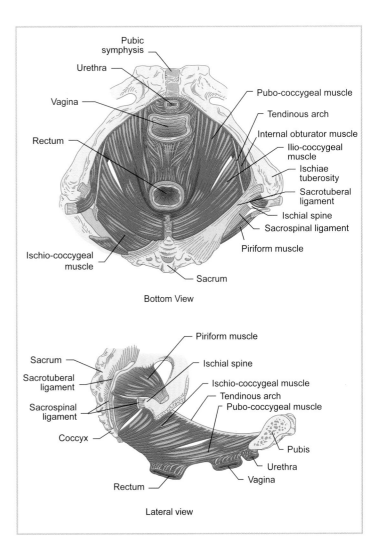

4.12 Pelvic diaphragm.

Simple
hysterectomy

PART 2

CHAPTER 5

Vaginal hysterectomy

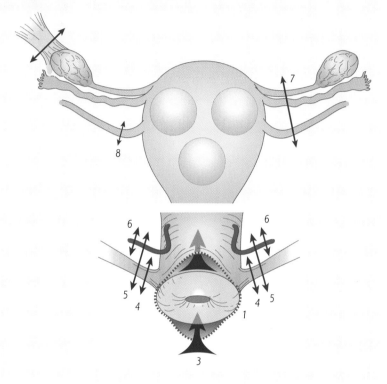

5.1 *Synoptical drawing.*
    1. Pericervical incision. 2. Vesicouterine dissection. 3. Opening of the Douglas pouch
    4. First passage of the Deschamps needle, uterosacral ligament. 5. Second passage of the
    Deschamps needle, uterosacral ligament and uterine artery. 6. Doubling of the uterine artery.
    7. Ovary conservation: ligature and section of the utero-ovarian pedicules. Adnexectomy:
    8. Ligature and section of the round ligament. 9. Ligature and section of the lombo-ovarian ligament.

Guide for the reader

1. To describe the successive surgical steps.
2. To identify the actions presenting a risk of inducing complications.
3. To state the measures to be used for the diagnosis and treatment of complications.
4. To precisely describe the conditions and surgical circumstances requiring a change to laparotomy.

Hysterectomy still remains the symbol operation of gynaecological surgery, and not without reason. On the one hand, despite the development of medications and conservative surgical techniques, hysterectomy is still the operation most frequently carried out on non-pregnant women. On the other hand, this operation retains a bad reputation among the patients as well as among numerous doctors. Since it is sometimes carried out too hastily, patients may feel that they have been "mutilated." Nevertheless, the great majority of these interventions are carried out for reasons of "comfort" in order to relieve functionally impeding disorders. In such cases, hysterectomy remains the last recourse among other treatment options of far less urgency. Reserved for cases for which more conservative methods fail, it will be experienced as a form of great relief by the patients.

Indications of "comfort"

A vaginal hysterectomy is not urgent if performed in order to relieve functional disorders.

Its advantages must outweigh the risk of the surgical procedure. It is used only for cases where more conservative methods have failed.

Prior to the operation, informed consent must be obtained from the patient.

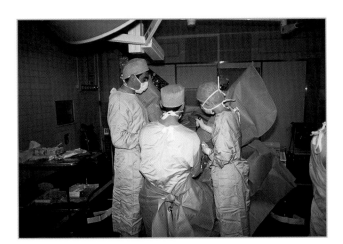

5.2 Positioning of the surgeon and his assistant surgeons.

With the development of laparoscopy and vaginal surgery, hysterectomy has become the symbol for the evolution and progress of gynaecological surgery. While a decade ago 80% of hysterectomies were still performed by laparotomy, this number has dropped to less than 50%, in some teams even to less than 10%. Daniel Dargent, who reintroduced vaginal surgery of the non-prolapsed uterus to France (never having been abandoned in other countries), was one of the main driving forces behind this development. This silent revolution has allowed the reduction of the mortality and morbidity associated with this intervention, as well as diminishing the costs (in comparison with laparotomy) due to shorter operating, hospitalisation and recovery times.

THE PRINCIPLE

The principle of this surgical procedure is to cut the suspending ligaments and install preventive haemostases from the bottom to the top, i.e., in the inverse direction relative to the process of abdominal hysterectomy (see *figure 5.1*). The procedure begins by ligature-cutting of the supporting ligaments of the uterine cervix, including the uterosacral ligaments and the paracervix (or cardinal ligaments). In the absence of a prolapse, the use of classical forceps, such as the Jean-Louis Faure forceps, is sometimes complicated by the narrowness of the operating field. We have, therefore, developed the habit of using Deschamps needles, which prove to be absolutely indispensable for vaginal hysterectomies on non-prolapsed uteri. Here we will describe the simple vaginal hysterectomy technique in the absence of a prolapse for a small uterus.

Similar procedures

Abdominal hysterectomy and its operational stages: for its mirrored operational pocedures and the techniques for suspension of the vaginal vault.

The techniques of myomectomy for the reduction of uterine volume.

POSITIONING AND PREPARATION

The preparation of the patient is minimal, with washing one day before the procedure, catheterisation at the beginning of the operation, and vaginal lavage on the operating table. Anaesthesia applied can be either general or loco-regional. If there is any doubt about the need for laparoscopic assistance, or if laparotomy might be required, it is advisable to notify the patient and to apply general anaesthesia.

The positioning for the execution of a hysterectomy is classical (*see figure 5.2*). It is advisable that the surgeon is sitting, while the assistant surgeons are standing on either side of him, each with sufficient access to the operating field to allow for surgical assistance with sufficient comfort. Ideally, the surgeon should work with two assistant surgeons as well as one instrument nurse. The sterilising solution is widely applied so as to allow the switch to abdominal hysterectomy if necessary.

DESCRIPTION

Sutures

Slow absorbable thread (type *Vicryl*, diameter 1) is recommended for vascular sutures, while for sutures of the ligaments or closure of the vagina, rapidly resorbing thread can be used.

Placement of the retractors and the Museux forceps

The operation begins by placement of lateral and posterior retractors, followed by the positioning of Museux's forceps on the anterior and posterior lips of the uterine cervix, respectively (*figure 5.3*). A firm tug on the uterine cervix now allows the assessment of uterine mobility and, consequently, the identification of possible difficulties that could be faced during the operation.

Infiltration

In the case of simple hysterectomy, a pericervical infiltration is not indispensable and must be discussed in view of possible anaesthetic contraindications affecting the comfort of the surgeon. The relatively weak bleeding that normally occurs during the operation essentially comes from the vaginal incision. This has the aesthetic and practical advantage that the use of aspiration and compresses can be minimised. Four infiltration points are identified (*figure 5.4*) , and the infiltration is applied to the outside of the blood vessels (verify by aspiration prior to injection) well below the vagina and not in its mass (*figure 5.5*).

Pericervical incision

In the case of preliminary infiltration, the incision is always pericervical, although the incision can be limited to the posterior part in order to reduce bleeding in the absence of

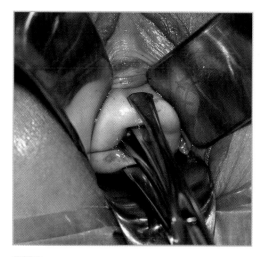

5.3 Museux's forceps on the neck of the uterus, with retractors in place.

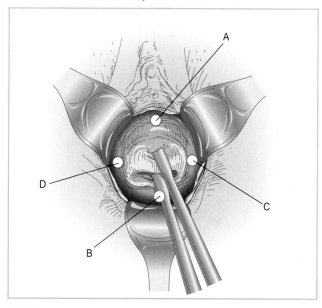

5.4 Identification of the four infiltration points.
A. Prevesical region (15 cc). B. Prerectal region (15 cc).
C. Left paracervix (5 cc). D. Right paracervix (5 cc).

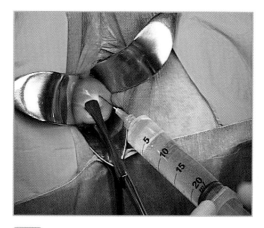

5.5 Anterior infiltration.

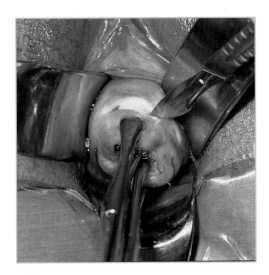

5.6 Deep anterior incision.

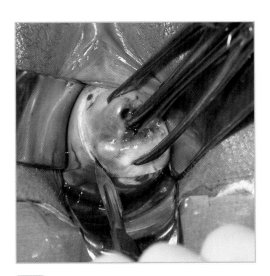

5.7 Superficial lateral incision

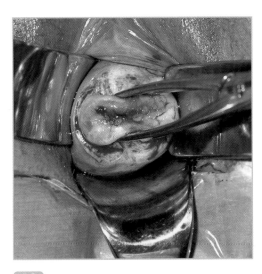

5.8 Museux's forceps grasping the edges of the incision.

preliminary infiltration. It is performed within the limit of the of the bladder's insertion onto the uterine cervix, whose bulging can be located just above the holding position of the Museux's forceps by releasing the pull on the neck of the uterus (figure 5.6). The incision is deep on the anterior and posterior segments, but laterally more superficial (*figure* 5.7). In fact, unlike during vaginal colpohysterectomy, the lateral parts of the uterine cervix are not dissected. On the contrary, the supporting ligaments of the uterine cervix are to remain attached to what will form the right and left parts of the vaginal incision at the end of the intervention. Ideally, these suspending ligaments are stiched laterally to the vagina during their initial ligature-cutting and again during the closing of the vagina.

Repositioning the Museux's forceps

The Museux's forceps can be repositioned by grasping the edges of the anterior and posterior incisions; They may be placed side by side, thus closing the uterine cervix and opening up the anterior and posterior dissection spaces by simple tension (*figure* 5.8), or they may be left on the individual edges.

Opening the Douglas' pouch

The fibres spanning the area between the front of the uterine cervix and the edge of the posterior vaginal incision (held by mouse-tooth forceps) are neatly cut (*figure* 5.9).

One can now view the Douglas' pouch by grasping it with forceps and folding it such that it arches into the dissection area. It can now be opened by quickly piercing it with scissors

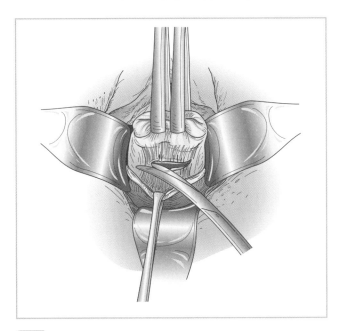

5.9 Opening the Douglas' pouch.

while holding it with dented forceps before enlarging it by opposing traction between the forceps and the closed scissors placed inside either side of the opening. The opening is completed by sliding a first finger in the place of one of the instruments, subsequently replaced by two fingers of the surgeon, which perform an outward motion. The posterior retractor can now be placed into the space created (*figure 5.10*) by oblique insertion before being securely positioned with a rotational movement. This insertion can be facilitated by leaving a finger in place for guidance and by placing the retractor at an angle of 45° laterally.

Difficulties in opening the Douglas' pouch

In case of elongation or posterior adhesion of the uterine cervix, or vaginal narrowness, difficulties can be encountered during the opening of the Douglas' pouch. It is sometimes necessary to search for the pouch higher up. In this case, one risks entering the uterine isthmus, which causes haemorrhaging, or a rectal wound.

A rectal examination can sometimes be quite helpful. If necessary, one can postpone this opening and first section the suspending ligaments, thus bringing the pouch towards the surgeon by increasing the uterine mobility. This section can either be carried out directly using bipolar scissors, necessitating a resumption when closing the vaginal incision, or following placement of the Deschamps needle. During this operational phase, a posterior retractor protects the rectum. Where persistent difficulties arise because of complete filling of the Douglas' pouch, one needs to know how to adapt to the situation by performing a diagnostic or even operational laparoscopy.

Vesicouterine dissection

After having opened the Douglas' pouch, the Museux's forceps are lowered in order to access the vesicouterine space. Due to the depth of the vaginal incision one can grip the edge of the vaginal incision with dented forceps in its median plane, just as done during opening of the Douglas's pouch. The sagittal connective fibres can be sectioned by stretching and subsequently performing a two centimetre long cut across their mid-point. Fine scissors, with their curvature pointing towards the uterus, are used to neatly cut the fibres at more or less 45° relative to the uterine isthmus before laterally enlarging the opening (*figure 5.11*). The dissection field now reveals areolar tissue replacing the sectioned fibres.

Here too one must identify the plane of dissection between bladder and uterus wherein a retractor can be placed in order to hold back the bladder. This is sometimes hard to find if coming too close to the uterus. Once the plane of dissection

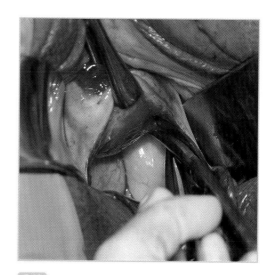

5.10 Douglas' pouch opened with a posterior retractor in place.

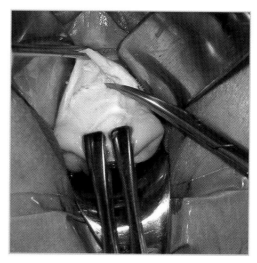

5.11 Beginning of the vesicouterine dissection.

Helpful techniques for locating and opening the Douglas pouch:

- vaginal palpatation
- rectal examination
- sectioning of the paracervix;
- diagnostic laparoscopy.

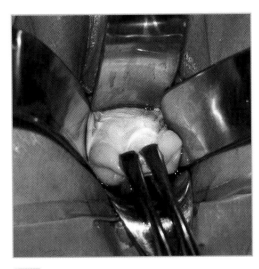

Placement of the anterior retractor.

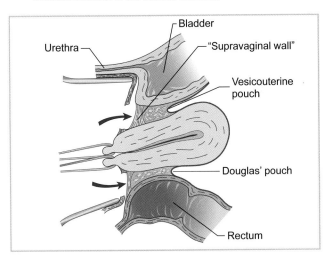

Opening the two peritoneal pouches.

Past history of Caesarean section

The principle of dissection of the vesicouterine space does not change. In most cases, the incision is situated higher up above the uterine isthmus because the uterovesical dissection will have been carried out for the abdominal approach. The dissection plane of the bladder's lower part, therefore, remains unaltered. It is advisable not to attempt the opening of the anterior pouch during the same operational stage, but to perform a secondary opening following establishment of the uterine tilt and the surgeon's exploration of the anterior pouch using his finger.

Locating the bladder

With even minimum experience, and in the absence of anatomical modifications, the locating of the bladder prior to performing the anterior cervical incision is not indispensable. If desired, this process can be simplified by partially filling the bladder, causing the anterior vaginal wall to bulge more obviously. Filling the bladder with a coloured liquid allows even very small wounds inflicted on the bladder during the intervention to be easily identified. Finally, in cases with a previous history of subvesical surgery or surgery due to vaginal malformation, one ideally places a Béniqué probe inside the bladder in order to visualise or palpate the vesical limits. However, it is our conviction that in the majority of cases such precautions are not necessary.

has been found, it can be easily enlarged by pushing back the bladder with a finger. Haemorrhages in this plane of dissection should not be present and would indicate rupture of the uterine or vaginal musculature. Likewise, it should not be adhesive unless there is a history of Caesareans. It is advisable to directly open the anterior pouch so that a retractor can be placed inside it during this stage of the procedure. This pushes back the bladder and, at the same time, removes the two ureters from the operating field, which becomes especially important during stages following ligature of the uterine pedicles. This opening is easily performed by experienced surgeons, but can be somewhat difficult in cases of a previous Caesarean (c.f. boxed text). However, even in such cases the space must always be correctly dissected allowing the placing of a retractor for holding back the bladder during later operational stages, even if it is not positioned inside the anterior pouch (figure 5.12). As for other retractors, this retractor must be handled with great care by one of the assistant surgeons who will not push it too far if the anterior pouch has not been opened so as not to injure the bladder.

Placement of the retractors

After opening the two peritoneal pouches (figure 5.13), the bladder and rectum are pushed back by the anterior and posterior retractors, respectively. The posterior Mangiagalli retractor is held in place by its own weight, but when placing

Encountering difficulties in the opening of the anterior pouch

For an experienced surgeon, the opening of the anterior pouch does not present any difficulties. However, where difficulties are encountered during dissection, or in the case of previous Caesarean, or even during apprenticeship of the surgeon, we recommend performing this opening after having established the uterine tilt as described in the above technique.

the Deschamps needle, is pushed further towards the back. The lateral retractors remain inside the lateral vaginal pouches, where they should not be placed too deeply. Even after ligature-section of the suspending ligaments and later of the uterine arteries, they must remain in this pouch in order not to damage or hide the pedicles.

Ligature of the paracervix

One can now perform the ligature-sectioning of the cervical suspending ligaments, which include the uterosacral ligaments (palpable by finger) and the paracervix. Traditionally one would now place clamp forceps, such as the classic Jean-Louis Faure forceps, but in the absence of a prolapse their use is inconvenient due to a lack of space. One will, therefore, prefer a Deschamps' needle equipped with a thread, with the thread held across about 10 cm of the needle's concavity and towards its convex part. In order to get hold of the complete paracervix in one go, one of the large pedicles needs to be pierced; here, the ligature might slide off, and it is, therefore, recommended to doubly secure it to assure homeostasis. The first passage of the Deschamps' needle is performed from the front towards the back, along a small fold that appears laterally, right above the uterine cervix, about 3 mm outwards, while the anterior retractor, always remaining in the median plane, holds back and protects the bladder and ureters (figure 5.14). One starts on the easier side. Before placing the Deschamps' needle, the uterine cervix is brought forward and the homolateral suspending ligaments are palpated by a finger slid into the posterior pouch (figure 5.15). This allows precise orientation of the Deschamps' needle in the antero-posterior plane, which is essential for the needle to pass well behind and not through the paracervix. As a result, this ligament, frequently large and located high up, can be gripped in a single effort. The needle is placed 5 mm laterally from and never in direct contact with the uterine isthmus, since this improves accessibility via the fold, and the needle can be passed without the need of excessive force. Requirement for the application of force when passing the needle indicates mis-positioning.

Recovery of the thread and suspending the vaginal angle

The point of the Deschamps' needle, directed by the surgeon's finger, pierces the broad ligament above the paracervices. The needle is pushed into the open Douglas's pouch, then slightly pulled back to relieve the tension on the thread which can now be gripped with dented forceps (figure 5.16). By pulling on the unthreaded end of the thread, the Deschamps needle can be removed. In order to attach the paracervix to the vaginal angle, the vagina wall is pierced twice across from the lateral vaginal incision (figure 5.17). The thread remains long and is

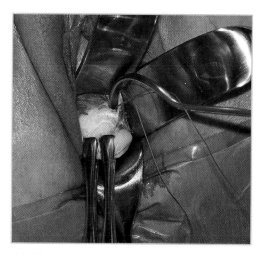

5.14 Anterior retractor pushing back the bladder and ureters.

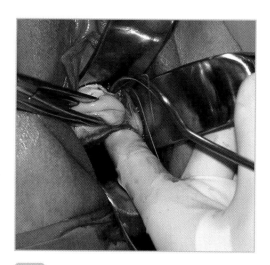

5.15 Palpating the suspending ligaments.

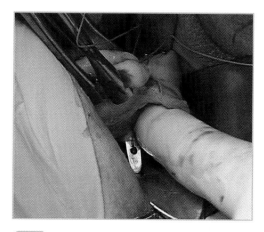

5.16 Grabbing of the suspending ligaments with the Deschamps' needle.

Limited uterine mobility

If difficulties are encountered when attempting to mobilise the uterus, arising from significantly thickened and retracted paracervices in relation with a constricted vaginal approach, these ligaments can be directly sectioned. This is done using either a cold scalpel followed, if necessary, by a secondary haemostasis, directly with an electrical scalpel, or even with other, unfortunately more expensive, methods, such as *Ligasure* or *Ultracision*. This procedure is only applied to the mentioned scenarios, since the secondary attachment of the uterosacral ligaments to the vaginal angles requires another operational stage in order to support the vaginal cuff. It is sometimes helpful to perform a partial section of the suspending ligaments, which will be completed after having thus improved uterine mobility.

fixed laterally in the operating field in case it subsequently slips off, requiring a repeat of the above procedure. Alternatively, it can be used for closing of the vaginal cuff at the end of the intervention. Now, a partial subtotal section of the ligament is performed (*figure 5.18*) before again passing the Deschamps needle. The section must increase uterine mobility without compromising the possibility of re-gripping the stump during completion of the knot. The sectioning must not be total in order to avoid injuring the uterine pedicle that has not been previously examined, and it is done perpendicular to the cervical axis where the thread has been placed. It is thus directly in contact with the cervix before running along parallel to it, favouring the posterior sectioning required to obtain the mobilising of the uterine cervix.

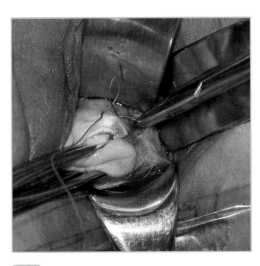

5.17 Attaching the paracervix to the future vaginal angle.

Second passage of the Deschamps' needle

In order to simplify the procedure and minimise the number of sutures, the second passage of the Deschamps' needle permits the reinforcement of the grip on the paracervix, and also provides a first hold on the uterine artery. It is helpful if the bladder and ureter have been sufficiently loosened from the uterus while performing the grip on the uterine artery or to complete such mobilisation at this point, so that the bladder can be pushed back (*figure 5.19*). In fact, it is the slight swinging motion of the anterior retractor that pushes laterally the pillar from the bladder and, as a result, the ureters that are included therein. In the great majority of cases, the uterine artery is visible if a hooked finger from behind correctly displays the broad ligament. In those rare cases when its viewing is not possible, the uterine artery can be palpated between the finger placed behind the uterine isthmus and the Deschamps' needle

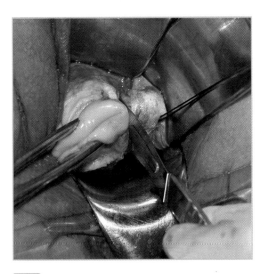

5.18 Partial section of the left suspending ligament.

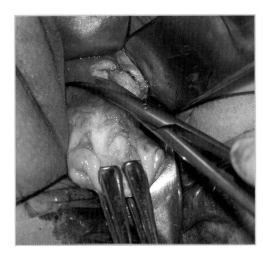

5.19 Additional vesical dissection when preliminary opening of the anterior pouch has not been performed.

placed in front. If necessary, the artery can be dissected, but palpation or viewing alone enable the locating of the uterine loop. The Deschamps' needle is then passed about 1 cm above its first passage inside this loop of the uterine artery (*figure 5.20*).

Finding the artery might prove difficult if it is very thin, if the tissue is thickened, or, in cases of cervical elongation, if there is, for example, the beginning of an hysterocele. One must, first of all, make sure that the bladder has been sufficiently dissected before placing the Deschamps' needle. While placing the Deschamps needle, just as during its first passage, one must ensure that the posterior grip on the paracervix is sufficient (*figure 5.21*). The thread is not threaded onto the needle, since no additional attachment of the paracervix to the vaginal angle is performed. The knot is tightened making sure that the whole of the paracervix is included. If need be, the paracervix can be gripped with Bengoléa-type forceps in order to pull it towards the median line, thus facilitating the inclusion of the whole paracervix.

Complete section of the suspending ligaments

Risk situations
At this stage of the procedure, two situations can present a risk factor:
– absence of an opening of the Douglas' pouch. Even if it is possible to grasp the uterine artery, this does not allow for increased mobility, and only ablation of a fibroma of the uterine isthmus, where present, would allow access to the peritoneal pouch. If the pouch is positioned high up, it can be located by palpation and subsequently opened after determining rectal location by a rectal examination. Endometriotic nodules of the rectovaginal septum that were not noticed, as well as dense adhesions of the posterior pouch will warrant doubts concerning the choice of surgical approach, which will now be more difficult, and present a risk of causing a major rectal wound. Diagnostic or therapeutic laparoscopy, or even laparotomy might prove necessary.
– total absence of mobility. This could be due to a large uterine volume, which sometimes prevents its descent into the pelvis. It might be desirable to perform a laparotomy following ligature-section of the uterine arteries, should this be possible by vaginal approach.

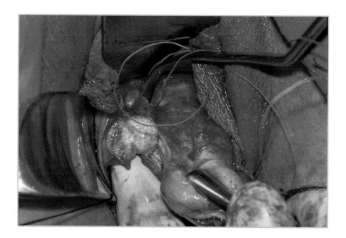
5.20 Second passage of the Deschamps' needle.

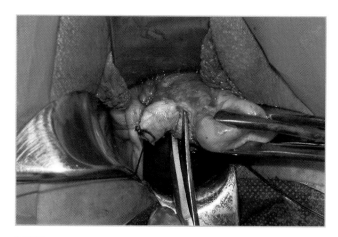
5.21 Completed section of the right paracervix.

The thread is cut short and one can now complete the section of the paracervix (*figure 5.21*). In the simplest cases, one can now dissect the homolateral uterine artery. In such cases, the Deschamps' needle would be passed counter-laterally as explained earlier for the sectioning of the paracervix.

Once the sectioning of the paracervices has been completed, the Douglas's pouch must be opened, if it has not been done at an earlier stage. Pulling on the uterine cervix usually brings it towards the vulva – absence of uterine mobility at this stage of the intervention represents an unfavourable prognosis for continuing with the vaginal approach. It can be verified by digital palpation whether sectioning of the suspending ligaments was complete and whether the peritoneum has been sectioned behind the broad ligament, the latter of which is often both necessary and helpful.

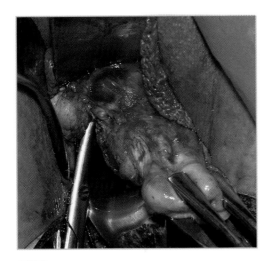

5.22 Dissection of the uterine artery.

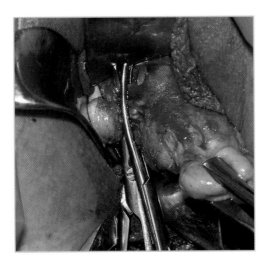

5.23 Grasping the right uterine artery with Bengoléa forceps.

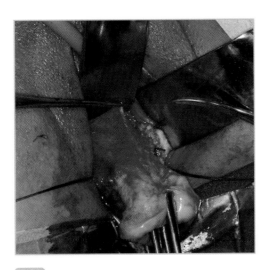

5.24 Revealing the anterior pouch.

Insufficient vaginal access

If uterine mobility is limited or vaginal access insufficient, succession of the operational stages is sometimes not possible. In such cases, a preliminary bilateral section of the two paracervices is performed.

Section and ligature of the uterine artery

In standard cases, it is easy to extend the paracervix' sectioning to the dissection of the uterine artery on either side. The uterine artery, already attached, must be doubled. The paracervix and posterior lamina of the broad ligament having been sectioned, one now extends the section ventrally by detaching the tissues covering the uterine artery; it can be made to stand out more clearly by sliding a finger behind it (figure 5.22). Naturally, the bladder must have previously been sufficiently freed. At this stage, the retractor is replaced under the bladder. The scissors are positioned under the uterine artery, which can be distinguished by piercing the tissues on both sides of the artery before opening the scissors' blades. Bengoléa's forceps can now be placed (figure 5.23) before sectioning the artery below the forceps' grip and suturing it with a thread that will double the first suture and that is cut short. The artery's visceral side does not require a ligature, since it only rarely bleeds.

Difficulties in performing the ligature

Following dissection of the uterine arteries, restricted vaginal access can hamper placement of the ligature. After having placed the Bengoléa forceps one can push the cervix back from the uterus in order to improve access to the uterine artery and facilitate passage of the finger to stretch the suture.

Uterine rotation

In typical situations the uterus will now be sufficiently mobile to allow its posterior rotation using Pozzi forceps. In the frequent cases where the uterus is large or vaginal access restricted, one will not be able to perform the uterine rotation without reducing uterine volume (c.f., Chapter 6 , "Techniques for reducing uterine volume"). Otherwise, rotation of the uterus will allow access to the anterior peritoneal pouch.

Opening the anterior pouch

Should the anterior pouch not have already been opened, this is now easily achieved (*figure 5.24 and 5.25*). After completing the uterine rotation, the surgeon's finger can be slid behind the uterus in order to bulge outwards the anterior pouch. The anterior pouch can safely be opened on the finger using scissors after rotation of the uterus (*figures 5.26 and 5.27*). Where uterine volume has been reduced during a previous procedure, viewing of the anterior pouch is facilitated by replacing the Museux's forceps on the uterine cervix. The opening is enlarged with scissors and the anterior retractor put into place before performing the ligature of the utero-ovarian pedicles.

Ligature-section of the utero-ovarian pedicles

In this Section, we concentrate on hysterectomies performed with the preservation of adnexa, annexectomy being discussed in Chapter 8.

The first stage consists in replacing the Pozzi forceps in cases of spontaneous uterine rotation, or the Museux's forceps in cases of previous uterine volume reduction. One forceps is placed on the uterine cervix, and the other is placed on the uterine floor across from the utero-ovarian insertion. Pulling on these two forceps stretches the homolateral utero-ovarian pedicle. One can now slide a finger behind this pedicle in

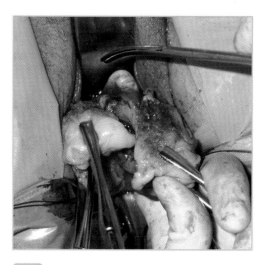
5.26 Anterior pouch displayed by the surgeon's finger.

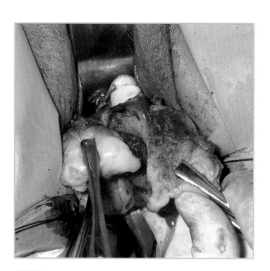
5.27 Opening the peritoneal pouch on the surgeon's finger.

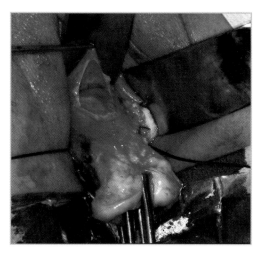
5.25 Opening the anterior pouch.

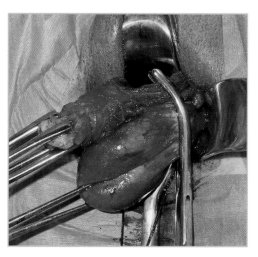
5.28 Clamp on the left utero-ovarian pedicle.

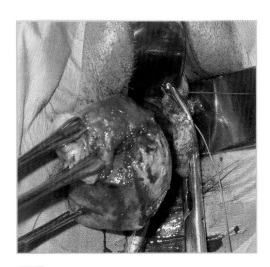

5.29 The utero-ovarian pedicle sectioned and sutured.

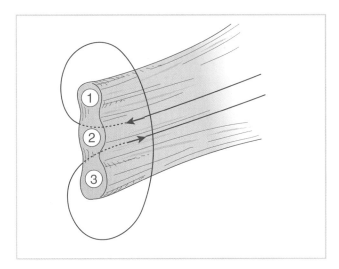

5.30 Heaney's stitch.
1. Round ligament.
2. Tube.
3. Utero-ovarian ligament.

order to test the pedicle's mobility and the ovarian integrity, and a clamp can be placed onto the utero-ovarian pedicle (*figure 5.28*).

The pedicle is consecutively sectioned from one, then from the other side so as to obtain uterine ablation. If the appendages are to be preserved, haemostasis of the pedicle must be assured. This often turns out to be a delicate manoeuvre, due to the pedicle's size that incorporates the utero-ovarian pedicle, as well as the broad ligament. To prevent the knot from moving following suture, we prefer performing this suture as follows: the thread is passed by transfixing the pedicle in its upper quarter before passing the thread above and over the top of the pedicle (*figure 5.20*), then passing around its circumference and transfixing the pedicle again in its lower quarter (*figure 5.30*). The thread is then knotted and kept long. This solid hold is further strengthened with spool suture (*figure 5.31*).

Occasionally the intestines can get in the way, and it might be necessary to place a gauze packing that holds back the small intestines during this haemostasis. The gauze is held by forceps and positioned progressively, and then it can be pushed back further by a retractor.

Controlling haemostasis and bladder integrity

With the gauze that holds back the intestinal coils still in place, haemostasis of each ligatured pedicle is verified. Bladder integrity is also verified during this operational stage.

In the case of long uterine morcellation necessitating successive anterior and posterior tractions on the uterus, the uterine ligatures must be examined carefully. Simple bleeding from the posterior vaginal incision or the base of one of the paracervices does not call for any specific action to be taken if

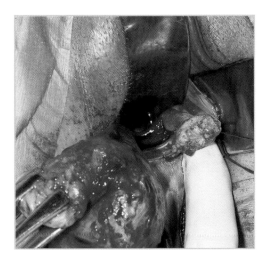

5.31 Folded utero-ovarian pedicle.

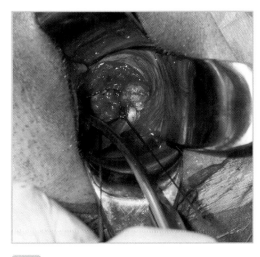

5.32 Pedicles sutured together in the left angle of the vaginal cuff.

the haemostasis is to be performed a second time during the closing of the vagina. In order to strengthen the vaginal cuff's secondary suspension and to diminish the risk of a subsequent prolapse of the vaginal fundus, the utero-ovarian pedicles and the suspending ligaments of the cervix are brought closer together by suturing (*figure 5.32*). If an annexectomy is performed, support of the vaginal cuff is obtained by bringing the suspending ligaments towards the round ligaments.

Detecting bladder injury: if in doubt about the bladder's integrity, especially after difficulties in opening the anterior pouch, one must be sensitive to any serous efflux during the course of the procedure. At this stage, one can easily inject 250 ml physiologic serum that has been coloured with methylene blue into the bladder in order to detect even the slightest vesical wound. Although one can avoid the more complicated cystoscopy, as suggested by many authors, to verify bilateral ureteral ejaculation, skipping this simple and rapid test may later be considered as a professional error if a bladder wound should subsequently be detected due to a uterovesical fistula.

Closing the vaginal cuff

Having performed all security measures and controls, one can now close the vagina after removed the gauze packing and having verified that the latter is not imbibed with blood from an unidentified haemorrhage. Since many studies have shown that a systematic peritonisation is not beneficial, we do not perform this technique for hysterectomies due to simple benign lesions.

In order to strengthen the vaginal angles' secondary suspension, the utero-ovarian pedicles and round ligaments

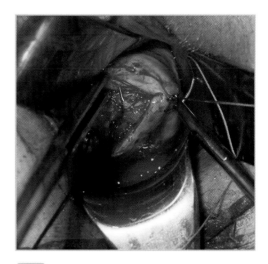

5.34 The left suspending pedicles are attached to the vaginal angle.

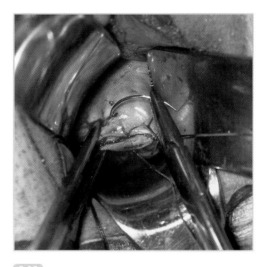

5.35 Continuation of vaginal closure.

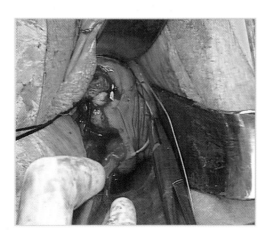

5.33 Start of vaginal closing.

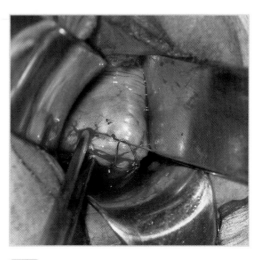

5.36 Crossed figure-eight stitches for vaginal closure.

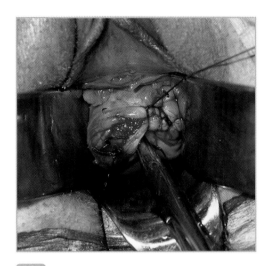

5.37 Connecting the right suspending ligaments.

of the paracervix are brought together at this stage. If the surgeon is right-handed the vaginal closure begins on the left by transfixing the vaginal incision externally to the paracervical pedicle, more precisely onto its lower and then upper part (figure 5.33); the stitch is knotted outside the pedicle and will represent the starting point of the closure. The paracervical thread that was kept long can be used for this stitch. The overcast stitch is continued, grabbing the lower part of the vaginal cuff, then transfixing the homolateral paracervix (*figure 5.34*) before taking the upper side of the vaginal cuff (figure 5.35) by crossing the overcast, thus bringing the suspending ligaments towards the vaginal angle. The overcast is continued on the vaginal cuff alone (*figures 5.36 and 5.37*), towards the opposite angle. Before reaching the angle, the suspending ligaments are tied as described (figure 5.38). The crossed overcast is terminated inside the cuff's angle, or on the counterlateral suture of the paracervix.

Placing a vaginal gauze drain is not necessary and only represents a source of vaginal infection. A urinary probe is not required, either, in the absence of an associated urinary intervention. Putting into place a catheter permits emptying of the bladder before releasing the patient from the operating room.

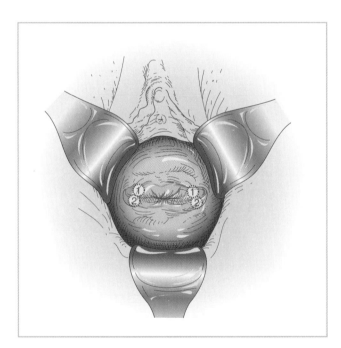

5.38 Final impression of the vaginal closure.
1. Utero-ovarian pedicle and round ligament.
2. Paracervix.

FOLLOW-UP AFTER THE INTERVENTION

Post-operative continuation:
− 48 to 72 hours hospitalisation;
− four weeks convalescence;
− no indwelling catheter;
− no vaginal gauze packing;
− weak metrorrhagia during one week, followed by leukorrhea for roughly three weeks;
− no sexual intercourse and no baths during one month.

Techniques for reducing

CHAPTER 6

Techniques for reducing uterine volume

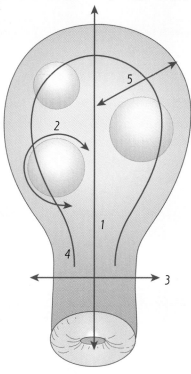

6.1 *Summary sketch.*
1. Hemisection. 2. Myomectomy. 3. Cervical section. 4. Endometrial coring.
5. Uterine morcellation.

Guide for the reader

1. To describe all procedures for the reduction of uterine volume.
2. To define the conditions required carry out this task.
3. To determine the advantages, disadvantages, and limitations of the procedures.

The techniques for uterine volume reduction have to be mastered so that even the most difficult hysterectomy cases can be performed, such as those with a high uterine volume (in our experience, a 100% reduction is to be performed where uterine weight exceeds 300 g) or those where vaginal access is limited. From our experience we conclude that these techniques are useful for over 50% of vaginal hysterectomies with benign pathology. Of course, such techniques are not advisable if there is risk of a neoplastic uterine process, the treatment of which would have to be decided preoperatively. The techniques for uterine volume reduction are easy to perform, but result in prolonged duration of operation, or even in increased bleeding during the operation. Apart from some exceptions, they have to be carried out after ligature-section of the paracervices and uterine arteries. Sufficient access to the uterine body is required. Thus, if the uterus is located above the promontory, or if the uterine body is impossible to mobilise, it is advisable instead to perform a laparotomy, thereby avoiding haemorrhagic procedures that will prove to be time consuming and rather inefficient.

All these techniques require mastery of vaginal surgery. They must be carried out progressively and under visual control, without excessive haste. Ripping or dilaceration of a vascular pedicle that could cause postoperative, sub-peritoneal bleeding can be prevented by exerting only moderate pull on the forceps. The assistants' retractors have to be repositioned at every new stage. This allows rotation of the uterus, as well as access to the anterior peritoneal pouch and utero-ovarian pedicles, by operational stages that might appear exaggerated in view of the overall uterine volume...

One usually refers to techniques for uterine volume reduction, since one technique alone is usually insufficient to bring about rotation of the uterus. Rather than the mastering of a single "miracle" technique, it is desirable that a solid strategy for uterine volume reduction be developed. The surgeon must never be caught unprepared; he must control the successive techniques for uterine volume reduction, the placement of the retractors by the assistant surgeons, and he must regularly regain his anatomical orientation by clinical examination. Thus, in our experience, we usually begin by uterine hemisection, terminated with a myomectomy or by morcellation of a

Precautions

A number of rules must be followed during the reduction of uterine volume:

- always work in the field of view;
- do not hurry and work methodically;
- regularly reposition the retractors;
- pay attention to the anterior pouch (if unopened), as well as to the bladder;
- do not pull excessively on the forceps;
- locate the utero-ovarian pedicles if the procedure moves away from the median plane.

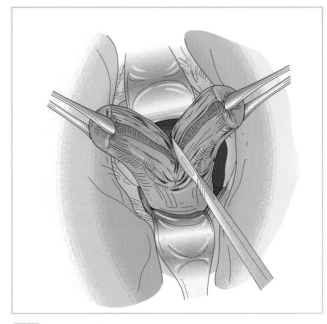

6.2 Hemisection.

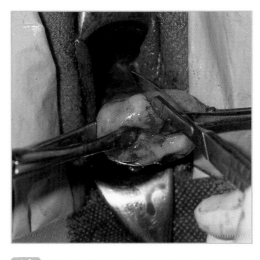

6.3 Beginning hemisection, anterior edge of the uterine cervix.

myoma. Where the uterus proves particularly large and, above all, if the myomas are located high up, it might be necessary to perform an anterior bisection or uterine morcellation in order to finally obtain uterine rotation.

HEMISECTION OF THE UTERUS

This is the first part of all procedures of reduction of uterine volume (*figure 6.2*). The Museux's forceps are repositioned on the uterine cervix by grasping its right and left parts, and tension is applied by one of the assistant surgeons. The anterior retractor is placed under the bladder in the peritoneal pouch, if opened at this stage of the procedure, and the Mangiagalli forceps are placed in the Douglas' pouch. The complete section of the cervical anterior lips (*figure 6.3*) is performed all the way to the upper part of the vesicouterine dissection using a cold scalpel, and then continued on the posterior lips (*figure 6.4*). The posterior incision is continued through the isthmus and uterus as far as the uterine mobility and vision permit. At this point, two more Museux's forceps are placed on the posterior edges of the incision (*figure 6.5*).

Tension applied to the two new forceps exposes another portion of the uterus, and hemisection can be continued (figure 6.6). This procedure is repeated until the full rotation of the uterus is achieved (*figure 6.7*). It might be necessary to release the uterine cervix in order to allow a better posterior tilt.

Two to three successive sections might suffice in the easiest cases to obtain rotation of the uterus. Nevertheless, in cases of

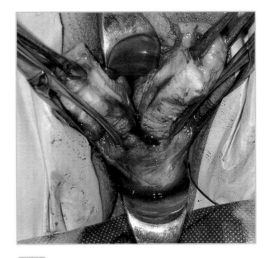

6.5 Placing the Museux's forceps on the edges of the hemisection.

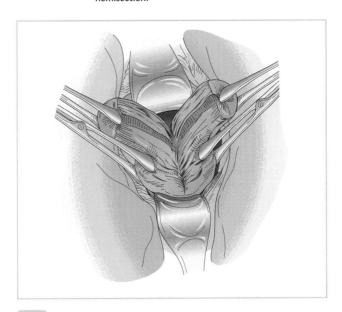

6.6 Continued hemisection.

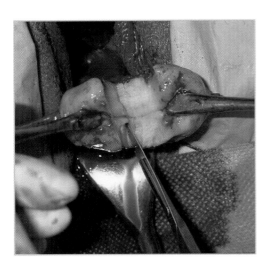

6.4 Hemisection of the uterine cervix.

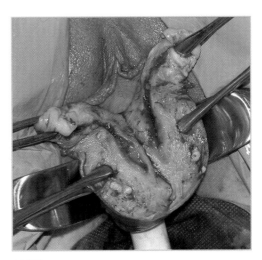

6.7 Complete rotation of the uterus following hemisection.

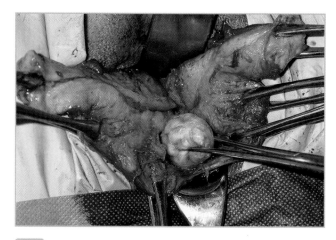

6.8 Myomectomy

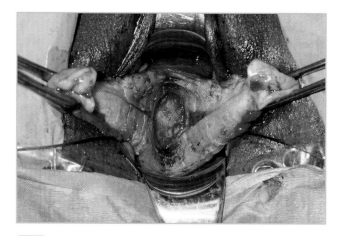

6.9 Fibroma visible at the limit of the bisection.

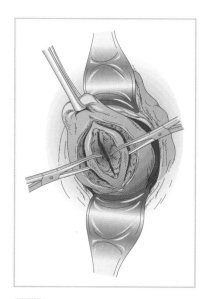

6.10 Primary myomectomy with bisection.

a larger uterine volume, a posterior hemisection may be insufficient and one reaches a point where posterior rotation will not be possible. Of course, if a partial posterior hemisection has already been performed to obtain access to a fibroma, it would be simple and efficient to now continue with a myomectomy. However, in case of a fibroma of the uterine fundus or of an anterior fibroma, it is necessary to interrupt the posterior hemisection in order to attempt progress on the anterior hemisection. The Museux's forceps are replaced on the uterine hemicervices and the cervix will be rotated posteriorly, exposing the anterior uterine wall and the anterior pouch. The latter will now be opened if it can be identified easily and if it has not already been opened at an earlier stage. After having protected the bladder by positioning the anterior retractor inside the anterior pouch, the hemisection can now be continued across the anterior uterine wall. This anterior hemisection is subject to the same rules as the posterior hemisection. It can provide access to anterior fibromas and in some cases even produce an anterior rotation of the uterus. Even when rotation does not prove possible, anterior hemisection often improves uterine mobility and allows returning to the posterior wall under improved conditions.

MYOMECTOMY

During the course of a hemisection, myomectomy represents an easy technique that is performed both rapidly and without danger, particularly if the fibroma's volume is but moderate (*figure 6.8*). Myomectomy is possible when the fibroma's inferior pole is visible or at least palpable (*figure 6.9*). If the fibroma prevents direct placing of a Pozzi forceps, one starts by partially bisecting the fibroma (*figure 6.10*). Pozzi forceps are the instrument of choice, since they are pointed, thus allowing a direct grip of the fibroma. A vigorous pull on the fibroma via the forceps is accompanied by a peripheral dissection performed with a finger of the other hand, thus allowing mobilisation of the fibroma. Removing of small fibromas is now easy. If the volume renders exeresis difficult, the fibroma will be morcellated.

MORCELLATION OF A FIBROMA

If the volume of a fibroma or the limited vaginal access do not permit the fibroma's direct exeresis, one starts by a partial hemisection of the accessible part. Museux's forceps are then placed on either edge of the incision to perform strong traction, and a peripheral dissection of the fibroma carried out as described above.

One will usually start with the most accessible part of the fibroma that has been freed by dissection with the help of a finger. Hemisection of the fibroma can then be enlarged, following the same rules as for uterine hemisection, or morcellation can be commenced (*figure 6.1*). Increasing the fibroma's mobility by dissection with the help of a finger is of utmost importance for hemisection of the fibroma. If the dissection can be performed entirely around the fibroma, its ablation is usually easy (*figure 6.12*). Should the dissection prove impossible, it is preferable to pull only on one side of the fibroma, thus exposing half of it. One then morcellates the visible part that is distally located from the Museux's forceps, making sure that the upper part is firmly held by replacing a forceps prior to completely sectioning the fibroma. This resection is ideally performed by successively working with quarters, as slices of an orange. If access to the fibroma becomes difficult, one can morcellate the fibroma's second half before performing a complete exeresis. This exeresis provides increased uterine mobility, thus enabling continuation of uterine hemisection or a new myomecty.

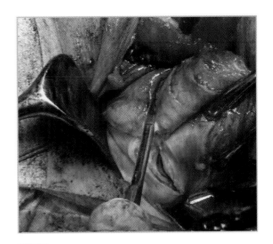

6.11 Morcellation of the fibroma.

UTERINE MORCELLATION

Certain fibromas are not accessible during an early stage and, in cases of moderate vaginal access, rotating a globally enlarged uterus is not always possible, even after hemisection. In such cases, one can perform uterine morcellation to reduce uterine volume, especially the uterine floor, (*figure 6.13*). One will ensure correct placement of the retractors and locate the adnexal pedicles. Uterine morcellation must always be carried out away from these pedicles, so as to prevent haemorrhaging during the operation. The two Museux's forceps are placed on one of the hemi-uteri, gripping the edge of the posterior hemisection. With traction applied, one dissects at a distance from the forceps, parallel to the hemisection's edges in "orange slices". The remaining part of the uterus is grabbed by two Museux's forceps and the procedure repeated as often as required. As a general rule, two successive ablations on either side are sufficient to markedly reduce uterine volume. One can now continue with posterior hemisection, or perform a myomecty if a fibroma has been detected during the course of the operation.

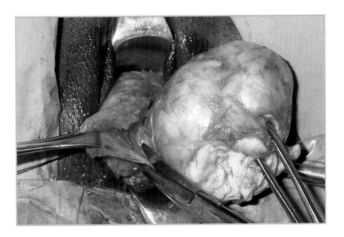

6.12 Final ablation of the fibroma.

ENDOMETRIAL CORING

Endometrial coring is an elegant technique for uterine volume reduction without the need of tractions or rotation of the uterine floor. Rotation of the uterus will be sufficient for a

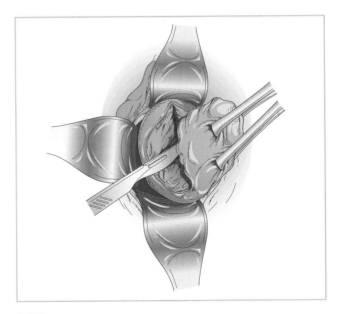

6.13 The myometrium is resected in quarters.

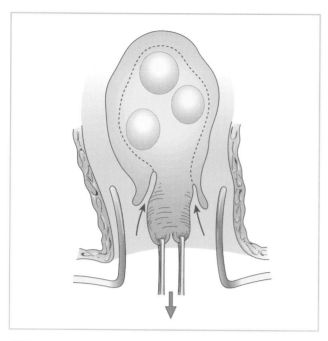

Endometrial coring; cross-section.

moderate uterine volume, but will not suffice with a relatively large uterine volume.

Elegance and limited haemorrhaging are the factors that give this technique its place in vaginal surgery. Furthermore, since it does not rely on the application of traction, it is especially well adapted for cases with adhesions of the uterine floor, which under these conditions do not risk of being torn during the procedure. The sketch illustrates the principle, and, especially, the cleavage plane applied between the myometrium's external third and its inner two thirds (figure 6.14).

Endometrial coring begins with a deep circular incision on the uterine cervix's base across from the uterine isthmus. One thus obtains access to the above mentioned cleavage plane, which is elongated using strong scissors while continuously pulling on the uterine cervix in order to favour the uterine removal (figure 6.15). The uterine curvature is followed while approaching the uterine floor for exeresis. The edges of the myometium's external third are again gripped with Museux's forceps and the uterus rotated, a procedure that proves much easier following the marked reduction in uterine volume. Opening of the anterior pouch and, more specifically, posterior adhesiolysis can now be performed under visual control.

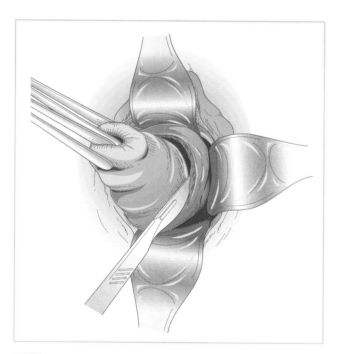

Initial circular supra-isthmian incision.

ADHESIOLYSIS BY VAGINAL APPROACH

If there is reason to suspect the presence of adhesions due to the patient's history or a clinical examination, it is advisable to envisage diagnostic or even therapeutic laparoscopy. The view obtained during an abdominal approach allows verification and treatment of dense adhesions of the uterine floor, possibly a pelvic endometriosis, that appeared after myomectomy. Where a Caesarian has previously been performed, the vaginal approach is both easier and less dangerous.

If adhesions are discovered during the course of the intervention, they can be treated via the vaginal approach under visual control. Unless the surgeon discovers a more serious situation than anticipated in this respect, which would have to be treated by laparoscopy or even by laparotomy, such adhesions can be dealt with during rotation of the uterus. Diagnosed by clinical examination during the course of the operation, the pelvic adhesions are treated according to appropriate security measures: by maintaining visual control, by sectioning with scissors, by not applying excessive traction, and by verifying the neighbouring organs.

Adhesiolysis by vaginal approach
Suspicion of major adhesions: laparoscopy or laparotomy.
Discovery during the course of the intervention: sectioning along the rotated uterus under visual control and verification of neighbouring organs.

AMPUTATION OF THE UTERINE CERVIX

Some surgeons prefer to precede uterine hemisection with amputation of the uterine cervix in order to facilitate the posterior rotation of the uterine floor, and thus the anterior rotation of the cervix and uterine isthmus (*figure 6.16*). Besides being moderately efficient only if the peritoneal pouch has previously been opened, loss of the two cervical halves for orientation represents the main drawback. This inconvenience is most marked in the case of long and difficult morcellation where the search for the anterior pouch is normally aided by applying tension to the uterine cervix.

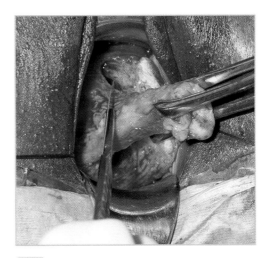

6.16 Amputation by section of the uterine cervix.

Once the uterus is rotated, one must not forget that the operation is not over. On the one hand, one has to verify the opening of the anterior peritoneal pouch, as well as the bladder's integrity, and on the other hand, verify homeostasis of the uterine pedicles that are sometimes endangered by successively pulling on the uterine cervix and rotating of the uterus. This verification is mostly typically carried out following ablation, because of the improved field of vision.

CHAPTER 7

Simple trachelectomy

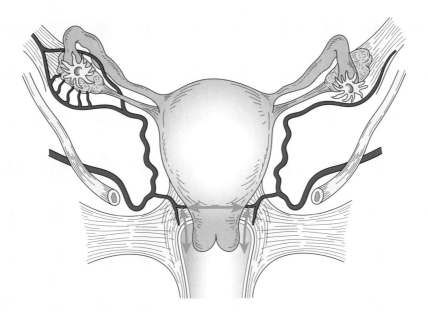

7.1 *Summary sketch.*

Guide for the reader

1. Rarely indicated, but its application is preferable by the vaginal route, clearly superior to all other routes of approach.

Simple trachelectomy is the term applied for two types of surgical interventions:
– a supravaginal amputation of the uterine cervix, which can be performed for certain types of micro-invasive cancer, followed by utero-vaginal anastomosis;
– a classical ablation of the remaining uterine cervix, as is still encountered due to the pointlessly persisting subtotal hysterectomy. Only the latter will be described, since it represents the archetypal procedure, best performed through the vaginal than by any other approach.

CASE DESCRIPTION

The case described is a recurrent *in situ* carcinoma on the remaining uterine cervix of a menopausal patient. This chapter is presented in the form of a report. A great many "tricks of the trade", which represent the main theme of this book, will be utilised.

ORDER OF OPERATIONAL STAGES

The operation begins similar to a simple complete hyster-ectomy. The remaining uterine cervix is grasped with forceps and firmly pulled towards the vaginal orifice (*figure 7.2*). Here, a trick frequently used in vaginal surgery is applied: a primary posterior incision (*figure 7.3*). Similar to abdominal surgery, this accentuates the mobility of the uterine cervix and allows better anterior access. Because above all, the natural adhesion to the

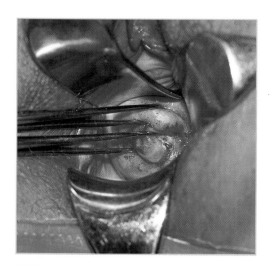

7.2 The remaining uterine cervix is held with forceps.

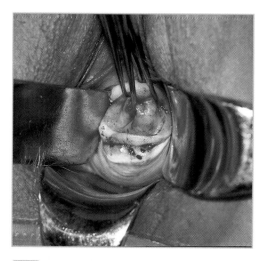

7.3 Posterior incision.

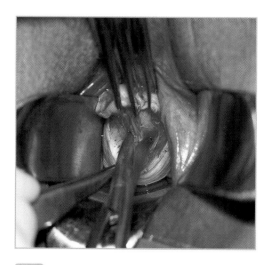

7.4 Access to the recto-vaginal septum.

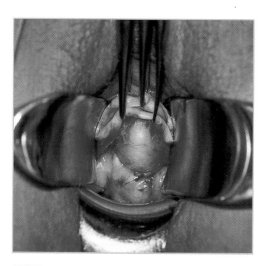

7.5 Opening the Douglas' pouch.

bladder poses a problem during simple trachelectomies. In the present case, one also notices an adhesion to the rectum which is treated similarly to the anterior adhesion to the bladder: the visible septum joining the vagina and the rectum is cut in the median plane, half-way between the incision's edges (*figure 7.4*). Further up along the posterior side of the uterine cervix we will find the Douglas' pouch (*figure 7.5*). It is located quite high up.

As expected, the anterior face is nicely revealed by this opening and posterior detachment procedure. An incision is performed in the anterior vaginal wall (*figure 7.6*). The two edges of the vaginal incisions are now available to be grasped with Chroback forceps, just as the vaginal cervix is held during a Schauta operation (*figure 7.7*). This grasp allows the lateral pouches to be revealed and incised (*figure 7.8*). The anterior detachment can now be completed following the already described method, which includes breaking through the supravaginal septum and obtaining access to the vesicouterine septum (*figure 7.9*).

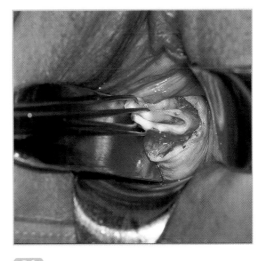

7.8 Lateral incision.

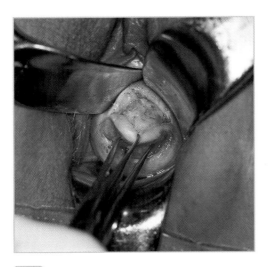

7.6 Anterior incision.

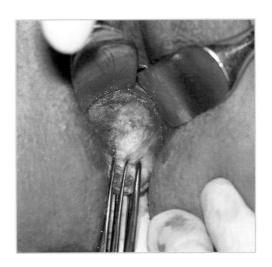

7.9 Completing the anterior detachment.

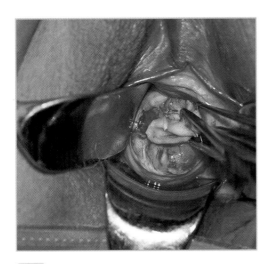

7.7 The vaginal edges are grasped with forceps.

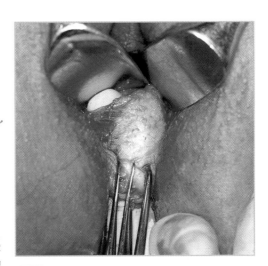

7.10 Opening the peritoneum in front of the remaining uterine cervix.

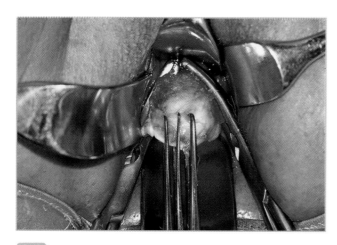

7.11 Forceps placed on the two paracervices.

One thus reaches the anterior peritoneal pouch. A finger can move from the Douglas' pouch to the anterior pouch (*figure 7.10*): the object has been circumscribed without risk to the bladder. The two paracervices are now grasped (*figure 7.11*), cut and attached.

ADVANTAGES

The patient may be released from the hospital the day following the operation.

In this case, no other approach is as efficient and safe as vaginal surgery.

CHAPTER 8

Annexectomy

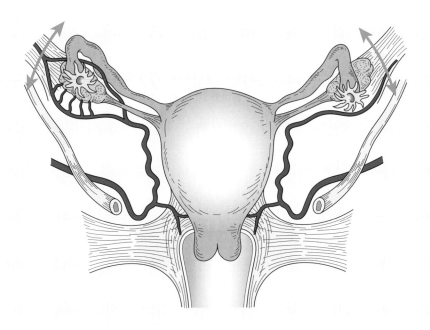

8.1 *Summary sketch.*

Guide for the reader

1. Any beginning vaginal surgeon will start with hysterectomy. The proportion of peri- or postmenopausal ovaries that the surgeon can remove during the course of the intervention is a good indication of his mastery of the route of vaginal access.

2. Furthermore, during a vaginal approach it is mandatory to respect the standards that have been established for the abdominal approach: any ovary that would have been removed during an abdominal approach must *a priori* be removed during a vaginal approach; surgery must always be adapted to the patient and not *vice versa*.

Vaginal annexectomy only makes sense if performed during hysterectomy. It is not always possible without the help of laparoscopy, especially in older patients with ovaries usually located higher up. It is particularly useful at the onset of the menopause in order to prevent ovarian cancers. However, we find that the majority of annexectomies are performed more frequently during abdominal as compared to vaginal hysterectomies: this is not acceptable. An alternative access route must allow all procedures performed via the access route of reference, which in this case is the abdominal route. In fact, beginning vaginal surgeons tend to refrain from oophorectomy, even though a specially adapted technique allows its performance via a vaginal approach. In particular, it is during hysterectomy, at the moment of the uterine artery ligature, when we determine the ease of removal of the majority of adnexae. (cf. boxed text).

Anatomical foundations of annexectomy: suggestions for success

1. The loop of the uterine artery is a characteristic point located between the descending parietal branch (originating from the hypogastric artery) and the ascending visceral branch (that joins the ovary and ovarian ligament). The artery must be clamped and cut at exactly this point, about 5 mm away from the uterine isthmus (*figure 8.2*) and not in contact with the uterus, in order to permanently separate the uterus and ovary from the lateral pelvic wall. If, on the other hand, both branches are clamped at the height of the isthmus, the ovary remains attached to the lateral pelvic wall and cannot truly be pedicled onto the lombo-ovarian ligament (*figure 8.3*). In contrast, elective sectioning of the properly identified (and perhaps dissected) loop of the uterine artery (*figure 8.4*) results in a complete detaching of the adnexa.

2. While the adnexa is being mobilised towards the center, the ureter remains in contact with the pelvic wall: if the adnexa has been separated from the wall, the ureter cannot be injured. Thus, this separation must be performed prior to this stage of the procedure (*figure 8.5*). To this end, the ideal site for taking hold of the adnexa is its "lateral pole", which includes the ovary's lateral pole and the tube structure: by taking hold of both, the ovarian ligament is efficiently stretched. If the adnexa cannot be mobilised, one has to switch to an abdominal approach or to use

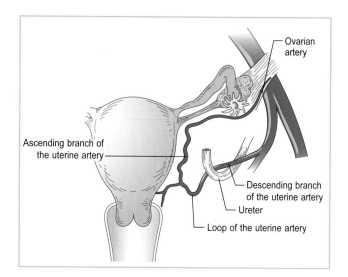

8.2   Loop of the uterine artery, the key to annexectomy.

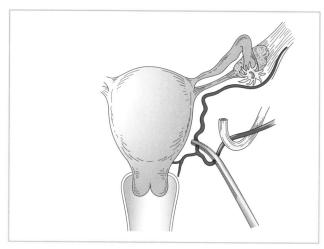

8.3   Incorrect techniquet: the loop is clamped twice, thus it will remain closed: after sectioning the pedicle, the ovary remains connected to the uterine artery.

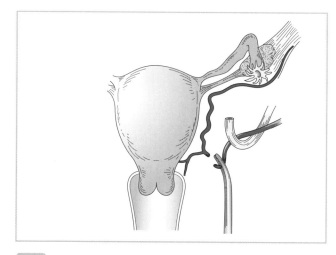

8.4   Correct technique: the loop has been opened and the adnexa completely pedicled onto the ovarian ligament.

laparoscopy (cf. paragraph "Laparo-preparation" in Chapter 10). For improved clarity, we show an abdominal view that illustrates this principle (*cf. also figure 30*.1 of the chapter "Visceral wounds"). The same grip on the adnexa, at the height of its lateral pole, must be performed during a vaginal approach (*cf. also figure 8.11*).

STRATEGY

The ovarian removals that are not possible via a vaginal approach, but nevertheless necessary, will be completed by laparoscopy after having completed conservative hysterectomy. In order to facilitate annexectomy, benign ovarian cysts can be punctured via the vaginal route as soon as their lower pole becomes visible. Cysts whose benign status is not certain should not be treated via the vaginal route.

Ovarian removal can equally be carried out with the uterus in place or following primary hysterectomy. If uterine anteversion is possible, clearly revealing the adnexae (hyperanteflexion is the best method to directly observe the adnexae brought into view and to identify the three elements inserted onto the uterine cornua: the tube, the utero-ovarian ligament in the back, and the round ligament in the front), it is advantageous to directly perform annexectomy (*figures 8.6 and 8.7*). In all other cases, one should start with the hysterectomy. The result is that the uterus will be replaced by two forceps, one placed on either utero-ovarian pedicle (*figure 8.8*). Alternatively, the above two approaches can be combined: if the adnexae are not directly accessible, the utero-ovarian pedicle is clamped and cut on one side only; this usually permits uterine anteversion and, consequently, access to the remaining adnexa.

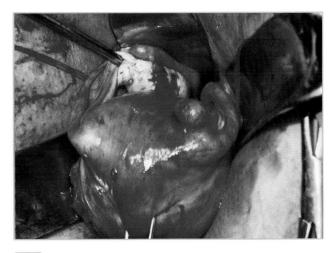

8.6   Observing the adnexae following uterine anteversion.

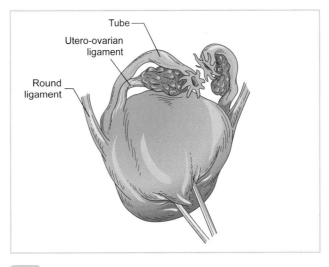

8.7   Observing the adnexa following uterine anteversion.

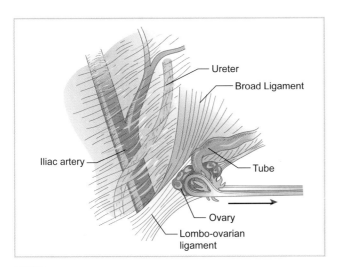

8.5   Bringing the adnexa towards the median line, if at all possible, separates the adnexa from the ureter and stretches the lombo-ovarian ligaments, leaving a large space for its clamping.

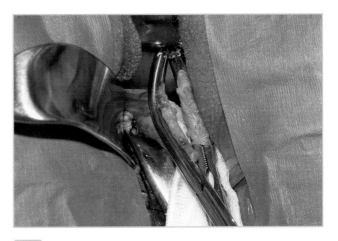

8.8   The adnexa following a first section of the utero-ovarian pedicles and hysterectomy.

OPERATIONAL STAGES

Vaginal annexectomy consists of six defined stages, whether the uterus is still in place (need for anteversion) or already removed.

– The three elements, round ligament (in front), tube (in the middle), and utero-ovarian ligament (in the back), are methodically observed (*figure 8.9*).

– As described earlier, the adnexa is pulled inwards using ring forceps, thus distancing the ovarian ligament from the pelvic wall and, consequently, from the ureter. The adnexa is ideally gripped at its external pole, in the region of the tubo-ovarian ligament: the ovarian ligament's distal part is thus directly brought forwards, all the while removing the potential obstruction presented by tube (*figure 8.10*).

– The round ligament is cut downstream of a strong forceps placed on its parietal stump. This section must be performed as far from the uterine insertion as possible: the more distal the section, the more direct the access to the ovarian ligament (*figure 8.11*). The forceps will be placed more distally, i.e. better placed, if the counter-lateral assistant exerts traction on the uterine fundus in the opposite direction, and if the homo-lateral assistant displaces the vagina as far as possible along the direction of the round ligament. The ligature of the parietal stump will be performed at the end of the procedure: the forceps, firmly held towards the pelvis' exterior by one of the assistants, helps with the displacement and contributes to the opening of the broad ligament, thus pointing the way to the ovarian ligament.

– The pedicled adnexa is now just attached by the ovarian ligament. All of its sides must be exposed. The median side is revealed by an adequate combination of a large retractor and

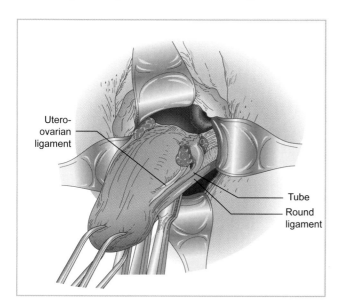

8.9 Left annexectomy (uterus in place): the cornua's three elements are identified: the tube, the utero-ovarian ligament, and the round ligament.

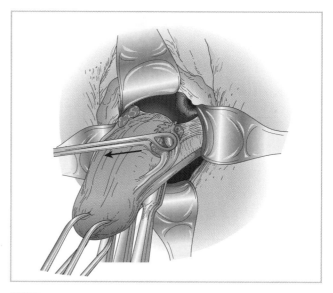

8.10 Left annexectomy (uterus in place): following uterine anteversion, the adnexa is viewed and grabbed on its lateral pole.

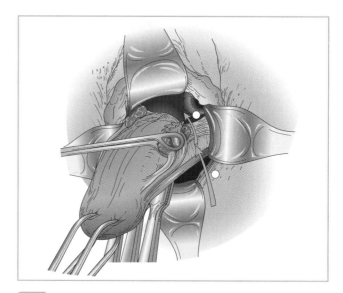

8.11 Left annexectomy (uterus in place): the round ligament is gripped as laterally as possible (arrow 1), so as to directly reach the ovarian ligament (arrow 2).

If the hold on the round ligament is not sufficiently distal, one must prepare the ovarian ligament by opening the anterior peritoneum and the cellular tissue of the broad ligament on the inside of the round ligament, to a point above the ovaries (*fig 8.11*).

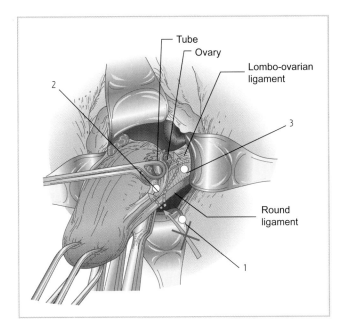

Tube
Ovary
Lombo-ovarian
ligament

2

3

Round
ligament

1

8.12 Wrong maneuver for sectioning the round ligament: too close
to the cornu (arrow 1). One comes too close to the cornua's
blood vessels (arrow 2) and has to incise the peritoneum from
the broad ligament's anterior wing in order to reach the ovarian
ligament (arrow 3).

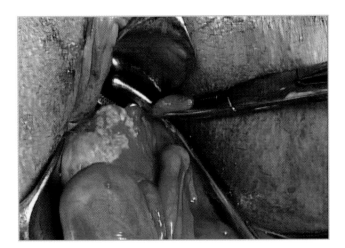

8.13 Left annexectomy, uterus in place. After sectioning the round
ligament, the appendage is merely held by the lombo-ovarian
ligament. A clamp, which should project beyond the pedicle, is
positioned onto the adnexa.

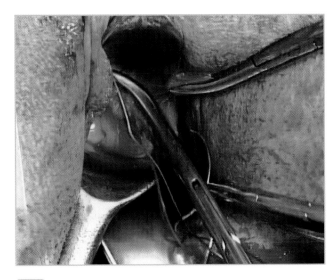

8.14 Left annexectomy. Ligature of the ovarian ligament, supported
along the upper and lower edges of the incision.

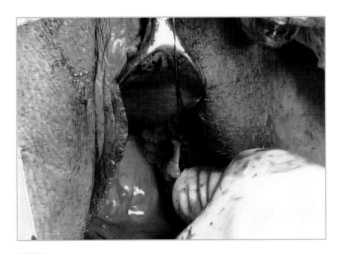

8.15 Left annexectomy. Final ligature of the round ligament.

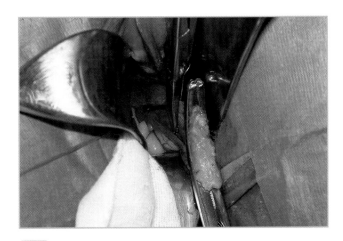

8.16 Left annexectomy following hysterectomy. One can see the
forceps that were used for a temporary haemostasis of the
cornua's pedicles. It is firmly pulled towards the outside and the
median plane. This is sufficient to reveal the ovary and to bring
out the round ligament for grasping. One can see the epiploic
fringes of the sigmoid.

a gauze strip holding back the small intestines. The lateral side
is also loosened as high up as possible using a Breisky retractor and haemostasis forceps. The lower side is viewed following sectioning of the round ligament and anterior leaf of the
broad ligament. The superior side must be viewed such that a
clamp, which should project beyond the pedicle (*figure 8.12*),
can be positioned without danger – one can thus delicately
perform the ligature. One makes sure not to have gripped any
neighbouring organ, then cuts.

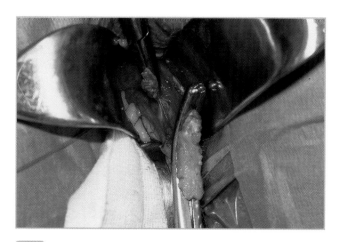

8.17 The round ligament is grasped and sectioned, the adnexa is connected to the wall merely by the ovarian ligament.

If hysterectomy is performed first, the first three stages are slightly, but not fundamentally, different. The first stage consists in taking hold of the adnexa lateral pole. The second stage consists in identifying the three elements of the uterine cornua, which can prove a little more difficult in the absence of the uterus. In case of difficulties, the easiest to identify is the tube, extended by its "ampoulla." The round ligament is in front, the utero-ovarian ligament at the back. The third stage consists of grasping (*figure 8.16*) and cutting (*figure 8.17*) the round ligament. The three last stages are identical, then the adnexa with or without uterus is removed by sectioning the ovarian ligament.

– The ovarian ligament is tied by a double ligature (*figure 8.14*), with crimping on both edges if access is sufficient, uncrimped (use a thread held by a long or thin forceps) if access is moderate, or using an Endoloop if access is limited. The threads are cut after having performed a definitive haemostasis so as to avoid any tractions.

– The round ligament is tied by stitching (*figure 8.15*).

Laparoscopic assistance

PART 3

CHAPTER 9

Laparoscopic assistance for the vaginal approach

Guide for the reader

The vaginal surgeon must also be a laparoscopic surgeon. The "academic" interest to master all three approaches – if one includes the abdominal approach – is of practical importance in many cases where the vaginal route proves dangerous or incomplete (cancers) or even simply impossible (fixed adnexae), but becomes reasonable for these cases as soon as the obstacle has been removed by a minimally invasive abdominal procedure. In fact, both approaches, vaginal and laparoscopic, require only moderate incisions: they are complementary, and not rival, techniques.

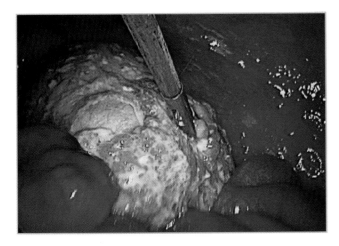

9.1   Ovarian cancer with exocystic growth.

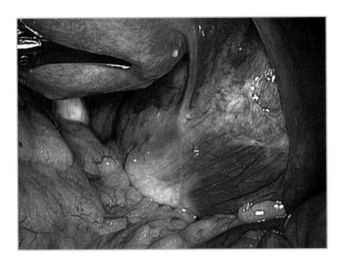

9.2   Benign ovarian cyst: no contradiction to a vaginal approach.
      It can be punctured by the vaginal route or simply removed
      together with the uterus, after laparoscopic preparation of the
      round and lombo-ovarian ligaments.

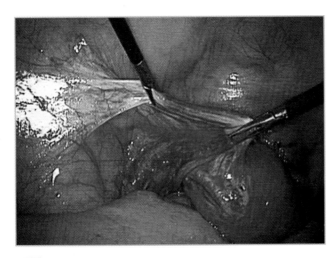

9.3   Individualisation of the left round ligament.

DEFINITIONS AND CONCEPTS

The concept of laparoscopicovaginal hysterectomy was born when it was understood that the two approaches – laparoscopico-surgery and vaginal surgery – could be complementary and not rival methods, the former permitting easier performance of the latter. The requirement to couple laparoscopy to a vaginal approach can depend on the surgeon's training (an assistance rate of 10% should not be exceeded: there are only very few indications for laparoscopic hysterectomies with ovarian conservation, while a number of ovarectomies can be performed by a vaginal approach) and the local conditions, the most important of which is a possible or certain pathology of the adnexae.

Strictly speaking, all laparoscopic hysterectomies are terminated by the vaginal route, thus justifying the generally applied Laparoscopically-Assisted Vaginal Hysterectomy (LAVH). However, the proportion of the intervention carried out by either the laparoscopic or vaginal approach may significantly differ, so this term is not particularly precise. Laparoscopicovaginal hysterectomy "à la française" is above all a vaginal hysterectomy, with the first operational stages performed by laparoscopy.

Laparoscopicovaginal hysterectomy, more than the laparoscopic imitation of an abdominal operation, is a tactical operation in its own right. It begins by laparoscopy and finishes by the vaginal route. The switch from one approach to the other is made when the vaginal approach is considered to be more efficient than laparoscopico surgery. This could be directly following an adhesiolysis, or after treating the upper pedicles. The decision depends on local conditions (including equipment and operating table) of the vaginal approach and on the practicability of laparoscopic maneuvers. Treatment of the lower pedicles can be entirely vaginal, or include laparoscopic sectioning of the utero-sacral ligaments, which can considerably facilitate a difficult vaginal approach. However, vaginal surgeons rarely treat uterine ligaments by laparoscopy (type 2 of Clermont-Ferrand), without even mentioning the extreme application of the laparoscopic technique by performing uterine extraction and vaginal suture laparoscopically.

Laparoscopy is interesting in that certain cases that are a priori difficult to treat vaginally may subsequently be handled via a vaginal approach. It also allows the identification of the best access route in the case of initial uncertainty. Three circumstances can be envisaged:

– primary laparoscopic diagnosis (type 0 from Clermont-Ferrand): diagnosis of an adnexal mass at the beginning of the intervention, verification that there are no massive pelvic adhesions and that the Douglas' pouch is not free allow vaginal surgery to be selected or, on the contrary, provide a contra-indication (figures 9.1 and 9.2);

– laparoscopicovaginal hysterectomy: pathologies of the adnexae or adhesions can be treated in order to facilitate or allow the intervention to be carried out by a vaginal approach; the question is when to switch from the laparoscopic to the vaginal stage; it is advisable to prioritise maximal efficiency and security and to laparoscopically treat pelvic adhesions, haemostasis of the ovarian pedicles, and, if need be, of the round ligaments (type 1 from Clermont-Ferrand) (*figure 9.3 and 9.5*). We keep for the vaginal approach that which is best done by this access: haemostasis and sectioning of the paracervices, of the uterine blood vessels, and of the utero-adnexal pedicles, and vaginal suture.

– conclusion laparoscopy: the end of vaginal hysterectomy can be marked by difficult access to the ovarian pedicle; if castration or haemostasis of this pedicle seem impossible by a vaginal approach, hysterectomy is completed via the natural access routes and a pneumoperitoneum created after vaginal closure, thus allowing oophorectomy and haemostasis to be performed (by coagulation or lasso).

PROBLEMS AND SOLUTIONS

Pelvic adhesions

If they do not fix together the organs, adhesions can be treated by the vaginal route. One must keep in mind that pulling on the uterine fundus or the adnexae can bring adherent intestinal segments downwards. These can easily be detached under the sole condition that the surgical view is satisfactory. A mobile intestinal segment accidentally injured can even be sutured during the course of the vaginal operation.

However, many postinfectious, postoperative, or endometriotic adhesions are not securely accessible via the vaginal route. They can prevent access to the uterine fundus or the adnexae. In such cases, laparoscopic preparation is highly recommended.

The order of events for adhesiolysis remains unchanged:
– freeing of the genitodigestive adhesions,
– identification of the ureters in cases of dense adhesions of the lateropelvic peritoneum;
– detaching the ovaries from the broad ligament's posterior side;
– isolating of the ovarian pedicles if oophorectomy is planned.

Each of these four stages must be detailed:

1. Freeing of digestive adhesions: one must merely clear those adhesions that hinder isolation of the genital tract before the procedure; those adhesions that hinder the laparoscopic view must not be cleared for this sake only; this illustrates the result of abusive laparoscopic assistance: clearing epiploic adhesions without clinical significance means losing time and taking unnecessary risks (*figure 9.6*);

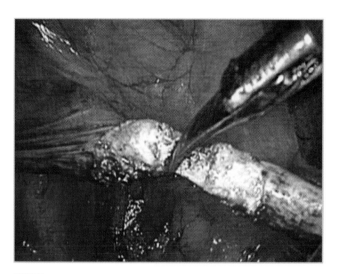

9.4 Sectioning (monopolar scissors) the left round ligament as far from the uterus as possible.

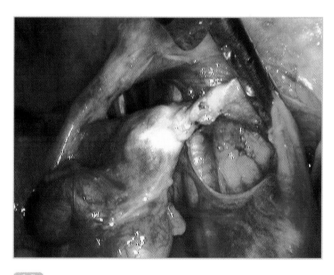

9.5 Coagulation of the right ovarian ligament, previously prepared by creating a window in the broad ligament.

Treatment of the vesicouterine pouch

It is not advisable to incise the anterior peritoneal pouch and to detach the bladder during laparoscopic preparation, unless a full laparoscopic hysterectomy is to be performed. It is not useful and even harmful. Such manoeuvres are more efficiently performed via the vaginal approach. It is, furthermore, rare to obtain the same cleavage plane during a vaginal approach, which means that, in any case, the work may need to be repeated during the vaginal stage. Even if this plane should be correct, an uterovesical detachment is more dangerous than helpful, since it modifies the conditions of lateral displacement of the bladder's pillar by the retractor placed inside the vesicouterine septum. Adequate lateral support of the bladder's pillar is the key to ureteral protection during vaginal hysterectomy.

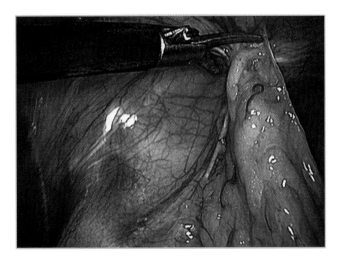

9.6   Clearing of adhesions.

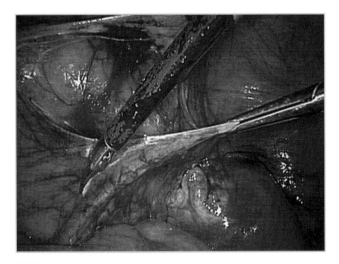

9.7   Lateral peritoneal incision outside the left ovarian ligament.

2.   Dense adhesions in the lateropelvic area represent a surgical danger for the ureter and may cause operative difficulties; such difficulties can be circumvented by a single manoeuvre of major importance, the lateral peritoneal incision (*figure 9.7*); an incision is performed perpendicular or parallel to the iliac vessels, i.e. very laterally and outside the region of adhesions, in healthy peritoneum; one will find the psoas major muscle, the iliac vessels, and the ureter (*figures 9.8 and 9.9*); no adnexal adhesions resist this simple technique.

3.   Liberating ovaries that are attached to the broad ligament's posterior side is easy if the adhesions are velamentous, and difficult if they are dense; dense adhesions must be liberated by an analogous gesture as that described for manual liberation in textbooks of classical surgery (*figure 9.10*) from the bottom towards the top, from the interior to the exterior, from the back to the front; this is done using forceps or an aspirator, replacing the fingers of a conventional surgeon; no section can be performed without exact knowledge of the ureter's path.

4.   The preceding stages are followed by individualisation of the ovarian ligament; an ovarian pedicle cannot be coagulated and cut until after having identified the ureter, or at the very least, until after the adnexa can easily be brought towards the median line; during difficult hysterectomies, identification of the ureter is highly advisable; it permits to create a peritoneal window between the ovarian ligament and the ureter, which allows secure coagulation of the pedicle; after the creation of the window and before any coagulation-sectioning, one has to verify that the ureter is located on the window's lower edge (*cf. figure 9.5*).

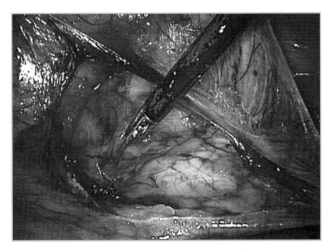

9.8   The iliac blood vessels and the sigmoid.

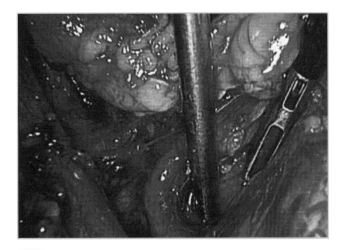

9.9   The hypogastric artery and the ureter.

Negative indications for laparoscopic assistance to vaginal hysterectomy

A history of Caesarean without complications or even iterative Caesarean, need for oophorectomy, nulliparity, and a large uterine volume are not in pricipal indications for a laparoscopic preparation. It has been proposed to consider pelvic pain as a decisive factor, since they could indicate an endometriosis or pelvic inflammatory; however, this argument is too weak if it constitutes the only element.

Myoma of the broad ligament

The myoma of the broad ligament is known as a potential operative difficulty, as well as a risk factor for ureteral lesions. Primary cleavage of the myoma makes both problems negligible and renders a potentially dangerous hysterectomy banal. In fact, in the majority of cases laparoscopic cleavage of the myoma is possible; this is not dangerous if the dissection plane remains strictly in contact with the myoma's capsule while performing the cleavage. This capsule must be accessed at the point where the myoma lifts the peritoneum from the broad ligament. Preparation of the cleavage is completed by a primary section of the ovarian and round ligaments. The myoma is now completely, or nearly, separated from the uterus: one can begin a standard vaginal hysterectomy.

Deep rectovaginal endometriosis

Here, the difficulty lies in the Douglas' pouch, sometimes at the height of the utero-sacral ligaments, less frequently laterally, close to the paracervices and up to the where the uterine artery crosses the ureter, and even up to the pelvic wall. It is often predictable by clinical examination, which must be complemented by an MRI, the only technique that shows the rectal wall's involvement. Oophorectomy is not a sufficient treatment for endometriotic nodules. If they prove symptomatic, one must, therefore, envisage their complete ablation. This is a long, difficult, and highly specialised procedure. Intestinal preparation must be perfect, since rectal injury, which can be sutured by laparoscopy, is not uncommon.

In all cases, there exist one or more spaces that should be exploited as during cancer surgery: the lower part of the rectovaginal septum, the paravesical fossae, and the pararectal fossae. The fossae (cf. chapter 4) are opened. The final goal of the rectovaginal separation is to gain access to the healthy rectovaginal septum.

Where there is a more or less sizeable nodule or merely a retraction of the fossae, there are exactly two options for initiating rectovaginal separation by laparoscopy: to pass either in front of or behind the nodule. Many specialists, especially

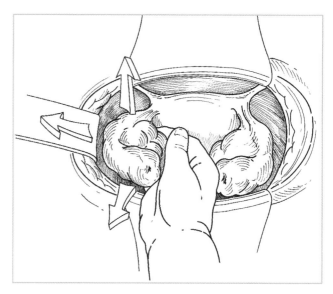

Traditional freeing movement: this is reproduced with the help of endoscopic instruments. (from "Techniques chirurgicales en gynécologie", by D. Querleu, 2nd edition, Masson, 1998)

those that have a CO_2 laser at their disposition (finding in this situation its last true indication) prefer to begin by a rectal liberation; this is by far the best option if one has to perform hysterectomy at the same time as removing the nodule. In difficult cases, it can be useful to commence by separating the nodule from the uterus, accessing the vagina (which has to be occluded by pneumostasis) and then completing the nodule's separation from the rectum.

Vaginal preparation of the rectovaginal septum

Beginning the operation by a vaginal approach can prove advantageous. The free part of the rectovaginal septum is directly accessible by this approach. The endometriotic nodule, once it has reached the vagina, is easier circumscribed by a direct incision. One rapidly obtains access to the adhesion between the nodule and the rectal wall, and this must be liberated as far as possible, an insufficient view being the only limit to the effort. One can sometimes completely liberate the rectum via this access route.

Cancer of the endometrium

Cancer of the endometrium can only be treated via a vaginal approach under two circumstances:
- Stage IA grade 1 endometrial cancer, where risk of dissemination to the lymph nodes is negligible and where a risk of tumor rupturing is non-existent;
- if the patient is generally in a mediocre state, counterindicating laparoscopy and laparotomy.

Laparoscopic lymph node dissection is no longer an investigational procedure

An experimental randomised trial has demonstrated that lymph node disection is carried out with equal comparable results by laparoscopy and laparotomy. Since the invention of laparoscopic lymphadenectomy in France, this technique has been widely adopted in numerous well-known centres throughout the world. It must be included in the repertoire of any surgeon treating gynaecological cancers. The technique must be as comprehensive as its open equivalent, with an average of 20 ganglions within the interiliac areas.

In consideration of the fact that lymph node dissection, the precise indications of which are, by the way, very controversial, can also be performed by laparoscopy, carcinoma of the endometrium should only be treated by a vaginal approach under the following two conditions:

– the successful ablation of the ovaries;

– the avoiding of any morcellation of the uterus, even if the literature does not show any data to support this rule.

If these two conditions are not met, the intervention can only be performed via the vaginal route if this is the only possible access route that can be considered, even in consideration of the imperfect circumstances, due to the patient being in a generally bad state. In such patients, treating exclusively by radiotherapy can also be considered. Generally speaking, these two rules should be respected, and laparoscopy proves helpful to this end.

Thus, the role of laparoscopy for surgery of endometriotic cancers is:

– lymph node dissection when indicated;

– haemostasis and section of the ovarian pedicles,

– uterine preparation for "atraumatic" hysterectomy, without excessive manipulation.

The last point is the most important. In fact, vaginal hysterectomy is often finalised by forced ante- or retroversion. Even though it is not shown that these techniques are linked to the recurrence of cancer, it is advantageous if they can be avoided, since they represent a potential cause of dissemination. "Atraumatic" hyterectomy may be performed laparoscopically by:

– sectioning the ovarian pedicles, as mentioned above;

– sectioning the round ligaments;

– incising the peritoneum on the broad ligament's posterior side, which, although not well known to anatomists, helps hold the uterus in place; the incision is performed, starting from the division line of the ovarian pedicles and ending at the cervical insertion of the utero-sacral ligaments, taking care not to injure the posterior uterine veins by incising the peritoneal wall (*figure 9.11*);

– if necessary, performing bipolar coagulation and sectioning of the utero-sacral ligaments.

Paradoxically, adding laparoscopy to a hysterectomy induces the risk of tubular backflow of tumour cells. Although the prognostic significance of this is not known, the risk has been shown to be related to the practice of intrauterine manipulation, which should, therefore, be avoided. To prevent this risk, one can occlude the tubes by coagulation at the beginning of the procedure.

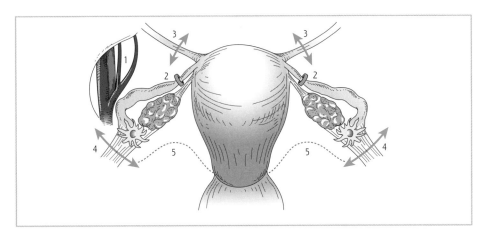

9.11 Laparoscopic actions for preparing vaginal surgery of endometriotic cancers.
1. Lamph node dissection (if indicated). 2. Coagulation of the tubes (at the beginning of all interventions to prevent tubal retrograde backflow of tumour cells). 3. Coagulation-sectioning of the round ligaments. 4. Coagulation-sectioning of the ovarian ligaments. 5. Incision of the broad ligament's posterior leaves.

Oncological surgery

PART 4

CHAPTER 10

The Schauta operation with preparatory laparoscopy

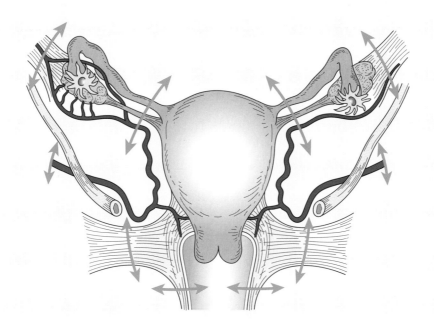

10.1 *Sectioning and haemostasis points during proximal-type radical vaginal hysterectomy.*

Guide for the reader

1. The Schauta operation is not an operation of historical significance. It is adapted for the needs of specific patients and has to become part of any cancer surgeon's repertoire. Mastering this technique forms the basis of radical trachelectomy.

2. Even if one is not led to perform the Schauta operation, practical knowledge of the ureter's anatomy is of great importance to a vaginal surgeon. The ureter can, and should, be palpated during all cystocele operations. During simple vaginal hysterectomy, the bladder's pillar, which contains the ureter, is protected by the retractors that are placed inside the vesico-uterine septum.

*T*he radical vaginal hysterectomy as described
by Schauta in 1901, modified by Stoeckel
in 1918 and Amreich in 1943 is known to only
few surgeons, since its mastery is difficult. In
trained hands, though, this surgical intervention
is of unrivalled elegance. It remains a highly
specialised operation, that must be performed with
"millimeter" precision: the wrong plane that causes
bleeding and hampers progress is often just a
millimetre away from the correct one. This intervention is just as radical as an abdominal approach
and is essentially performed on patients where prior
irradiation does not form part of the treatment. Its
only drawback is not to include lymph-node dissection, and it has, therefore, only taken on novel
indications since the development of endoscopic
surgery. Extraperitoneal laparoscopic lymph-
node dissection has been performed by Dargent
since 1986, and Querleu and Leblanc performed
transperitoneal laparoscopic lymph-node dissection
in 1988: in 1991, the combination with Schauta's
intervention lead to the development of a new concept that we have termed "Schauta's intervention
with laparoscopic assistance". By referring to the
French term "coelioscopie" used for laparoscopy,
Daniel Dargent coined the term "coelio-Schauta"
in the year 1992.

ANATOMY

Radical surgery is a treatment for uterine cervix cancers that
have not reached the pelvic wall. It is essentially composed
of removal of the paracervix or cardinal ligaments, the distal
parietal parts of which is a vasculo-nervous and lymphatic
structure, while their visceral proximal part is more fibrous in
nature. We will continue to call these structures paracervices
in order to respect the international anatomic nomenclature
Nomina Anatomica, and avoid the name "parametrium"
wrongly used by many authors. All radical hysterectomies
(abdominal, vaginal, laparoscopic, laparoscopically assisted
vaginal) are based on the knowledge of the surgical anatomy
of the paravesical and pararectal fossae, which are separated
by the paracervix, the removal of which defines radical
hysterectomy (*figure 10.2*).

The relations of the uterine artery and the ureter are well
known for the abdominal approach, but these are seen
differently during a vaginal approach. On the one hand,
the anatomy is viewed as reflected by mirror in relation to

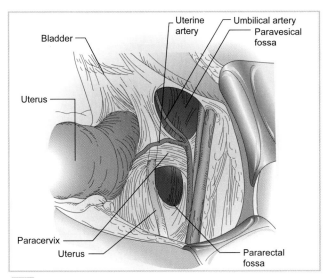

10.2 Essential anatomic elements for radical hysterectomy.

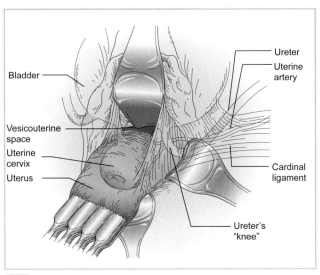

10.3 Anatomy of the ureter inside the bladder's pillar.

Definitions and indications

Radical hysterectomies, whether abdominal, vaginal or
laparoscopic, can be classified into two categories:

– distal hysterectomies (type III or Meigs operation), fully
removing the complete cardinal ligament;

– proximal hysterectomies (type II or Wertheim), removing
the median part of the cardinal ligament that is perpendicular
with the ureter, inside the emergence of the lateral vesical
ligament ("anterior parametrium").

Proximal hysterectomy is the modern version of radical
hysterectomy, used for exclusive surgery best indicated for
the treatment of early cervical cancer: grade IA2 and IB1
tumours, preferably with a diameter of less than 2 cm. The
operation described here corresponds to the proximal version.

an abdominal approach, and on the other hand, traction applied on the uterine cervix at the beginning of a vaginal intervention alters their interplay by drawing down the ureter to a point known as its "knee", the lowest point of its descent (*figure 10.3*).

LAPAROSCOPIC PREPARATION

Lymph node dissection

Diagnostic lymph node dissection is performed on the "inter-iliac sentinel area", defined by the space between the external and internal iliac arteries. This concept is only applicable with cervical cancers than are smaller than 4 cm, where the probability of a skip common iliac or aortic metastasis is low. Realisation of lymph-node dissection requires opening of the paravesical fossa, and it is useful to also laparoscopically open the pararectal fossa (*figure 10.4*).

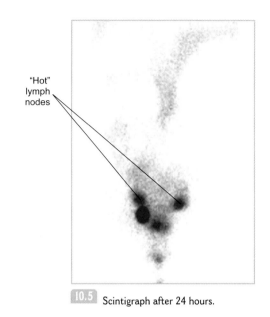

"Hot" lymph nodes

10.5 Scintigraph after 24 hours.

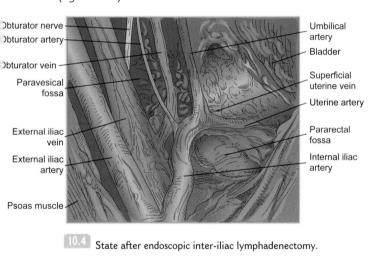

Obturator nerve
Obturator artery
Obturator vein
Paravesical fossa
External iliac vein
External iliac artery
Psoas muscle

Umbilical artery
Bladder
Superficial uterine vein
Uterine artery
Pararectal fossa
Internal iliac artery

10.4 State after endoscopic inter-iliac lymphadenectomy.

Removal of the sentinel lymph node, identified by the intracervical injection of a patented blue stain or of isocyanine blue (or even of an isotopic marker), is a procedure that is still under investigation (*figures 10.5 and 10.6*).

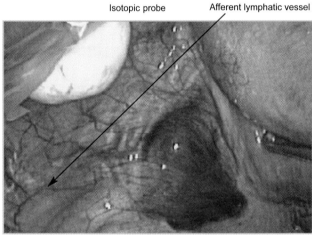

Isotopic probe   Afferent lymphatic vessel

10.6 Laparoscopy with identification (blue and isotopic) of the sentinel lymph node.

Sectioning the uterine artery and the superficial uterine vein

The beginning of the uterine artery is freed during lateropelvic dissection. It is found at the ventral part of the orifice entering the pararectal fossa (*figure 10.4*), and is isolated over 1 to 2 cm, just like the superficial uterine vein that runs along it (*figure 10.5*). Both are coagulated (bipolar coagulation) and then sectioned (*figure 10.7*).

Following this action, the uterine body is separated from the pelvic wall, but the cervix remains naturally attached to the

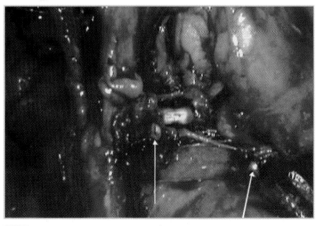

10.7 The uterine artery is sectioned following bipolar coagulation. The superficial uterine vein has been coagulated.

paracervix, the cephalic edge of which becomes visible (*figures 10.8 and 10.9*).

Section of the upper pedicles

The round ligaments are coagulated and cut. If required, this gesture will facilitate forward rotation of the uterus during the vaginal stage. The ovarian pedicles can be treated during the vaginal stage. In case of oophorectomy, it might be helpful to do this during the laparoscopic stage. However, where the adnexae are to be preserved, laparoscopic treatment of the utero-ovarian pedicles is not useful.

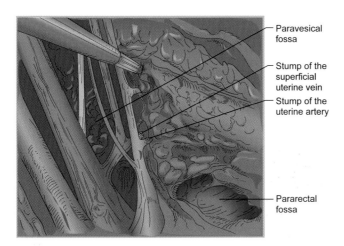

Paravesical fossa

Stump of the superficial uterine vein

Stump of the uterine artery

Pararectal fossa

10.8 State after sectioning the uterine vessels.

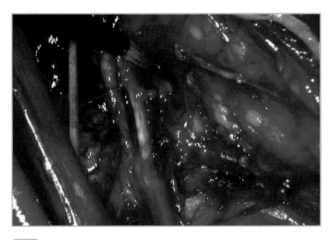

10.9 State after sectioning the uterine vessels.

VAGINAL OPERATION

General strategy
The idea is to incise the vagina at an adequate height in order to produce a vaginal collar, to open the paravesical and pararectal fossae, and to then identify and dissect the ureter before grasping the paracervix.

Generally speaking, there is no need of perineotomy to perform this surgical intervention. In cases where the vagina is extremely narrow, we advise a laparotomy. If narrowness of the vagina's internal orifice renders vaginal access difficult, a limited median episiotomy can be helpful without resulting in postoperative pain or disturbing scars.

Making vaginal cuffs

The vaginal cuff is constituted by a circular incision that is generally positioned 2 cm from the cervical insertion or at least 2 cm from the lesion. Make sure not to remove too much of the vagina, easily done in the posterior pouch, which is much softer and deeper. The anterior and posterior incisions are easier to perform than the lateral incisions, since the lateral fornices are shallow and difficult to access. Therefore, one ends with the lateral incisions either immediately, or after having grasped the collar's median part with Chroback forceps (cf. infra), which allows application of firm traction to expose the lateral fornices. During all stages of the incision the retractors are indispensable for exposing the incision line.

The vaginal wall is pulled forward by Allis' or Kocher forceps, which are placed directly inside the chosen incision line, with six to eight forceps being placed in a circle (*figure 10.10*). Traction applied on these forceps produces a evagination of the vaginal wall. At the summit of this evagination, between the two vaginal layers thus pulled forward, one will inject adrenaline-containing lidocaïne (if the anaesthetist contra-indicates the use of adrenaline or even of lidocaïne one will use physiological serum). Mechanical detachment, supplemented by the haemostatic effect, will help to identify this plane during separation of the vaginal cuff.

The incision concerns the entire thickness of the vagina's external layer. Presence of the liquid infiltration indicates that the incision has been neither too deep (the deep layer, which is part of the operative piece, must not be involved) nor too superficial (one would not be able to access the rectovaginal and vesicovaginal septa) (*figures 10.10 and 10.11*).

The vaginal wall is gradually put under tension from the circular progression of the incision by the traction on individual forceps combined with the application of tension using a retractor situated across from it. This incision concerns all of the external wall of the evagination both in the front and in the back. Laterally it is less deep, so as to maintain the cervix' lateral attachments for the vaginal collar. To facilitate this lateral incision, it might be helpful to wait until having completed the subsequent stage on the median line, in order to profit from the traction on the vaginal cuff.

The vaginal cuff is turned inside out and closed with five to six Chroback forceps, which enclose the tumour inside the upper third of the vagina (*figures 10.11 and 10.12*). The operative specimen can now be pulled and oriented by one of the assistant surgeons.

Stages on the posterior zone

Logical succession of the operative stages

We elect to commence with stages on the posterior zone that allow the lowering of the operative specimen before carrying out those on the anterior, which gives the following order: opening of the Douglas' pouch, opening of the right pararectal fossa, section of the right uterosacral ligament (defined by the two previous openings), opening of the left pararectal fossa, section of the left uterosacral ligament, opening of the left paravesical fossa, detachment of the left ureter, opening of the right paravesical fossa, detachment of the right ureter and, finally, treatment of the vascular pedicles (paracervix, then upper pedicles, or upper pedicles, then paracervix).

The Douglas' pouch is revealed by pulling the vaginal cuff upwards with the help of Chroback forceps. The pouch is opened widely with scissors towards the uterus' dorsal side (*figure 10.13*). In order to open the right pararectal space, two Kocher forceps are placed on the vagina's edge, one at 9 o'clock the other at 8 o'clock positions. The entrance to the pararectal fossa lies between these two forceps and is revealed exactly on the vagina's deep side by applying axial traction on the forceps. The scissors break into the fossa, deepening it towards the ischial spine. The rectovaginal ligament is defined as the structure located between the Douglas' pouch (opened with a Mangiagalli retractor) and the pararectal fossa. The thus defined ligament is nothing other than the uterosacral ligament's rectovaginal part (*figure 10.14*). We will cut this ligament either on the fly, between two forceps, or using bipolar scissors – we always choose the last option. One thus obtains access to the recto-uterine part, which lies deeper, and where the section along the lateral peritoneal side of the Douglas' pouch will have to be completed. One must take care to cut only as far as one can see (the retroligamentous ureter is not far). Section of the broad ligaments' posterior leaflets is extended as far up as possible. This will mobilise the operative specimen and free the dorsal side of the right paracervix,

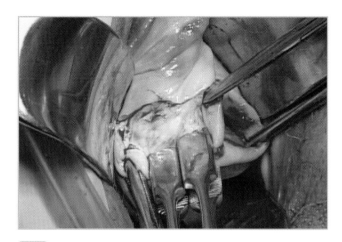

10.10 The vaginal incision.

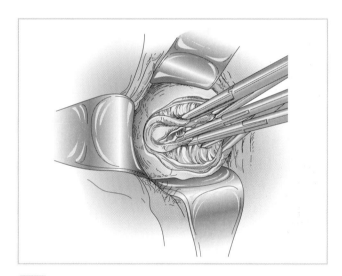

10.11 The vaginal incision.

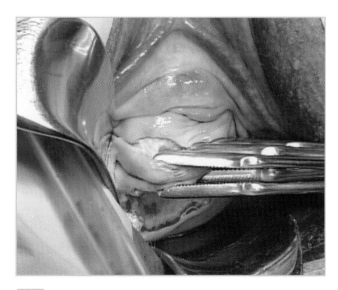

10.12 The Chroback forceps put into place.

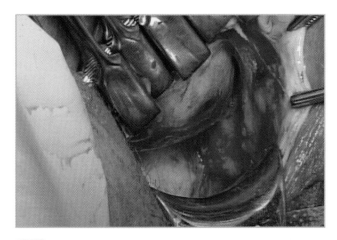

10.13 Opening of the Douglas' pouch.

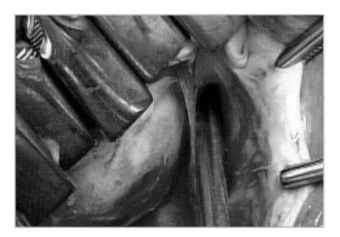

10.14 The left pararectal fossa is opened with scissors.

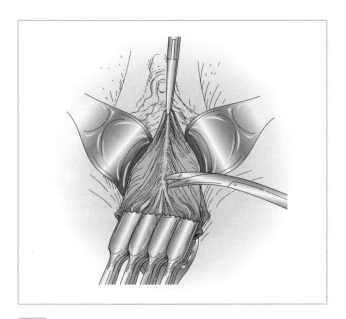

10.15 Opening of the vesicovaginal septum.

which can be palpated for reassurance. The same action is symmetrically repeated on the left hand side. Usually, this procedure does not permit the ligaments' complete sectioning; later, this will finally be handled by sectioning their uterosacral lateral part.

Ventral stages: opening the vesico-uterine septum

A firm traction on the Chroback forceps now orients the specimen downwards. Thanks to the posterior mobilisation, the anterior part of the operative zone is better visible. The goal is to prepare the vesicovaginal space, with special focus on the bladder, which, pulled downwards by attachment to the vaginal section, forms a larger recess than during simple complete hysterectomy, due to a larger dissection. As during standard vaginal hysterectomy, the fibers linking the bladder to the vagina's deep side must be cut between these two organs, closer to the uterus than the bladder, but not within the uterine fascia (*figure 10.15*). The vesico-vaginal and vesico-uterine spaces, and, finally, the characteristic peritoneal fold of the anterior pouch are thus reached.

The delicate moment
Dissection of the bladder represents a delicate stage of the surgical intervention. Only an experienced vaginal surgeon will be able to recognise the finest fibres oriented sagittally among the many fibres located between the bladder and uterus; these represent the entry to the vesico-uterine septum. Taking a wrong path will, of course, result in bladder injury. Installing a rigid orBénique's probe sound inside the bladder permits a vaginal surgeon in training to reliably identify this organ before and during the section. Wrong paths inside the uterine fascia are more frequently taken and more insidious: they hamper correct identification of the bladder's pillar and render later operative stages for the ureter's identification extremely difficult.

The vesico-uterine space must be widely opened towards its top and sides so as to reach the broad ligaments: easy execution of this action indicates a good detachment (any difficulty or bleeding indicates a wrong path). The action is neither complete nor correct if the uterine arteries' loops are not visible within the broad ligaments, on the right and on the left of the uterine isthmus: in fact, the vesico-uterine space laterally communicates with the broad ligaments (*figure 10.16*).

Ventral stages: opening the paravesical fossae

The procedures for opening the paravesical fossa, for dissecting the ureter, and for sectioning the paracervices will only be described for the left side. The same procedures will be symmetrically applied on the right side.

The ureter is located inside the bladder pillar (cf. figure 10.3), which is defined as the tissue between the paravesical fossa and the vesico-uterine space. The vesico-uterine space is already opened. In order to work in the left antero-lateral zone, the Chroback forceps are oriented in the diametrically opposite direction, i.e. downwards and towards the right. The paravesical fossa orifice is situated slightly in front of the radius located at 3 o'clock, exactly on the vagina's deep side. Two strong forceps are placed on the vaginal section, at 2 o'clock and 3 o'clock, respectively, in order to reveal this orifice (figure 10.17). Radial traction on these forceps indicates a groove into which the closed scissors are forced while keeping them in contact with the vagina's deep side. If the scissors are placed correctly, they should be "swallowed" by the paravesical fossa and the procedure should be bloodless. The scissors' smooth entry is only disturbed, at about 5 cm of depth, upon reaching the crossing of the aponeurotic insertion on the levator muscle. The scissors will be opened in order to enlargen this aponeurotic orifice. Subsequently, they will be replaced by a finger that will move forcefully into the fossa, palpate the ischiopubic branches, and free the bladder's lateral side all the way to the pubis ventrally and the ischial spine dorsally. First a thin, then a broad Breisky retractor will be placed inside the trench; this will reveal the lateral side of the bladder's pillar (figure 10.18). Since the vesico-uterine space is already open and, consequently, its medial side already freed, the bladder pillar is now totally visible.

Ventral stages: dissection of the ureters

The ureter is located inside the bladder pillar. At this point of the surgical intervention, it is impossible to differentiate the "internal" part (vesico-uterine ligament) that is medial to the ureter, from the "external" part (lateral vesical ligament or "anterior parametrium"), which is located laterally to the ureter and is not yet visible. The pillar's vesical insertion (close to the forceps) is close to the ureter's end, and traction on the vaginal collar, the uterus, the uterine artery and the vesico-uterine ligament will bring the ureter towards the surgeon. Key to the ureter's identification is its palpation between a finger placed inside the vesico-uterine space and the retractor placed inside the paravesical fossa. The finger is placed at the deep end of the vesico-uterine space and crooked, pointing towards the outside.

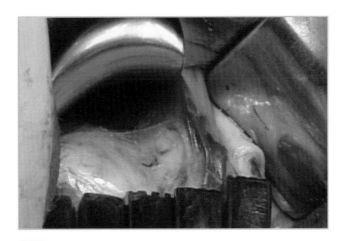

10.16 A retractor is placed inside the vesicovaginal fossa.

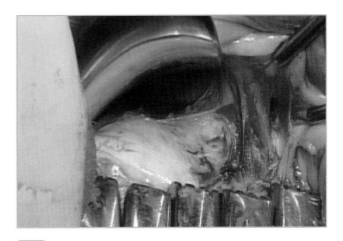

10.17 Opening the left paravesical fossa.

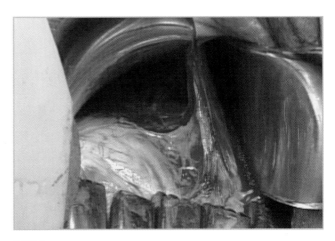

10.18 Opening the left paravesical fossa.

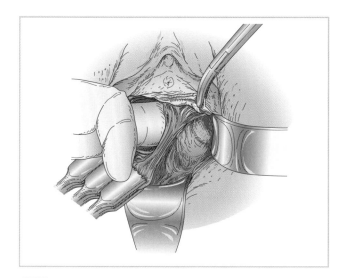

10.19 Palpating the left ureter.

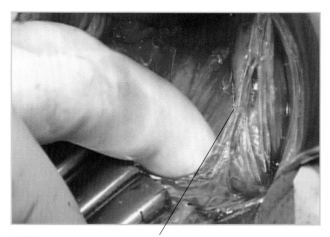

10.20 Locating the left ureter.

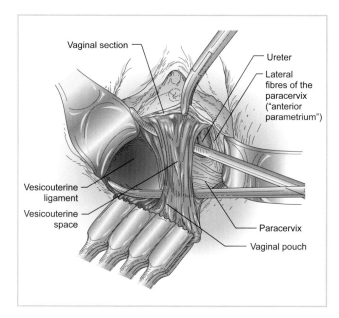

10.21 Defining the caudal fibres of the bladder pillar (left side).

It will run along the bladder pillar, pressing it against the retractor (*figure 10.19*). A bulge or even a noise (a characteristic "pop" or "click" sound) indicates the ureter's knee and its two adjacent segments, one ascending towards the bladder, the other descending. In easy cases, one can even visually perceive the ureter on the pillar's lateral side through the transparent lateral fibres once the finger has been placed inside the vesico-uterine space and pushes laterally against the bladder pillar.

Once the ureter has been palpated or seen, the lower side of the ureter's knee must be freed by sectioning the pillar's most distal connective fibres (*figure 10.20*). One can apply either of three techniques:

– the oldest consists of displaying the bladder pillar with the help of a finger placed inside the vesico-uterine space and then sectioning with a scalpel the lateral fibres opposite the ureter.

– the second consists of perforating the pillar below the ureter's knee with the help of an angled dissector, moved from the pillar's lateral to its medial side; the branches are separated below the ureter's knee and the thus prepared fibres, which are nothing else but the vesico-uterine ligament, are then cut (with bipolar scissors or between two ligatures). This technique is ideal if the ureter's knee is directly visible inside the pillar (*figure 10.21*); this action can be facilitated by grasping the pillar's distal part with a Babcock forceps, which pulls forward the fibres that are to be delimited.

– the third technique consists of dividing the bladder pillar with scissors, starting at its lower edge until the ureter becomes visible; the medial "internal" fibres, ureter, and lateral fibres are thus delimited; one must take especial care not to damage the lateral fibres, since they contain the bladder's nerves; a dissector is first passed behind the medial fibres, below the ureter's knee, and then the dissector is opened. One has to pinch or cut with bipolar scissors away from the uterus (*figure 10.22*), taking care with the vesical corna: we are now close to the ureter's entry into the bladder.

Treatment of the paracervix and upper pedicles

Delimitation of the paracervices
The paracervix has two sides and two edges. The anterior face has just been revealed during liberation of the ureter, while the posterior side has been prepared during section of the rectovaginal and recto-uterine ligaments. The paracervix' lower edge is attached by the paracervix' paravaginal segment (paracolpos). The upper edge is delimited by a fibreless zone inside the uterine isthmus, below the uterine artery's loop: this represents the "para-isthmic window" (figure 10.23).

There are two possibilities to treat and clamp the paracervices. Treatment from bottom to top follows the preceding actions directly without having to reposition the retractors or the uterus. Treatment from top to bottom, on the other hand, can be performed if uterine anteversion is carried out in a Doderlein manoeuvre. This manoeuvre is facilitated if the round and, in case of castration, lombo-ovarian ligaments have been treated by laparoscopy.

Treatment from top to bottom

This stage is essential to the intervention. Whenever possible (this is not always the case) we will choose the technique that consists in first opening the anterior peritoneal pouch from one round ligament to the other, in taking hold of the uterine fundus and performing its forced anteversion (Doderlein technique: *figure 10.24*), while diminishing traction on the vaginal cuff. Some additional forced anteversion is now possible and the uterus is held merely by the lower pedicles. As the operative field opens up, the ureter becomes visible. Where possible, this technique provides an excellent view of the uterine arteries and the unsectioned part of the uterosacral ligaments, as well as on the cardinal ligaments, which are pulled by the traction onto the operative specimen. The uterine arteries' ascending part, which follows the direction of the uterus, can now be clearly distinguished from their descending part (*figure 10.25*). It is drawn towards the operative field, thus allowing progress above the ureter's knee, as far as its origin, which has been coagulated and cut.

Forced externalisation of the uterine fundus becomes more and more intense, perfectly revealing the uterosacral ligaments' part that has not been treated at the beginning of the operation. It is now cut both on the right and the left with bipolar scissors, away from the uterus. The uterus is now merely held by the cardinal ligaments. At this stage, they can be clamped at a desirable position before being attached (*figure 10.24*).

Treatment from bottom to top

This is the other option. The paracervix' lower edge is defined by the vagina's separation from the paracolpos (*figure 10.26*). After these actions, the left paracervix is thus freed on all sides. One can grasp it. The objective of all preceding

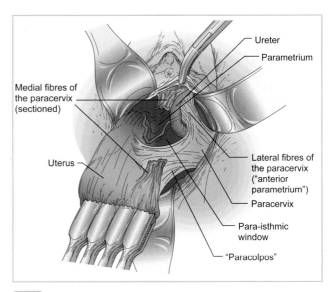

10.23 Situation after sectioning the left vesicouterine ligament.

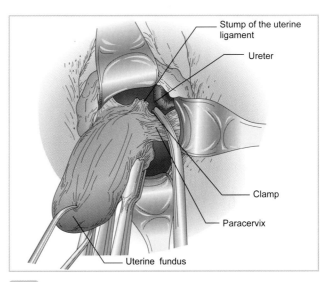

10.24 Treatment of the left paracervix from top to bottom (Doderlein maneuver).

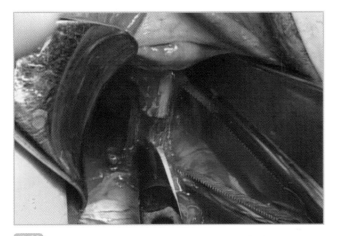

10.22 Section of the caudal fibres of the bladder's left pillar.

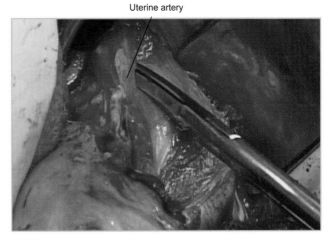

10.25 "Repatriation" of the left uterine artery.

74

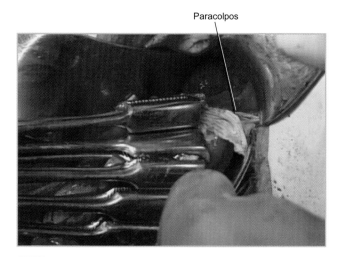

10.26 Identifying the left paracolpos (transversal ligament).

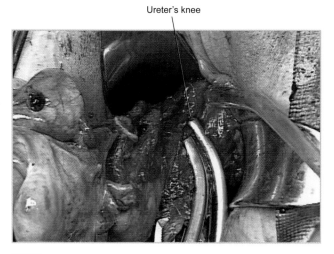

10.27 Section of the left paracervix: ureter's knee.

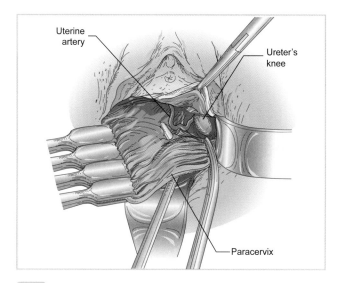

10.28 Paraisthmic window.

operative stages was to perform this step without risk. A Rogers' forceps is placed on either side of the desired point of section, i.e. immediately beneath the ureter's knee (*figures 10.27 and 10.28*).

A first clamp is positioned, which will draw a longer portion of the paracervix towards the operative field and will allow the more lateral positioning of a second clamp. After cutting, the parietal stump will be tied. Of course, all these actions will be performed first on the left and then on the right hand side. The cardinal ligaments' ligatures will be kept long and the needles threaded for subsequent use (cf. infra). It is common that some uterosacral attachments remain following this gesture. They will have to be sectioned with bipolar scissors or between two forceps: the uterus is now merely attached by its upper pedicles.

Opening the vesicouterine pouch, ligature and section of the ovarian or utero-ovarian pedicles and round ligaments, section of the broad ligament's and fibrous tissue's posterior side are often-associated, standard procedures.

Terminal stages

Peritonisation is not needed. If one has taken the precaution to prepare haemostasis of the posterior uterine veins, which tend to bleed after removal of the uterus, drainage is not required. This can be done by using the threaded needle kept from the paracervices' ligature. This allows reinsertion of the cardinal ligaments on the vagina, taking all tissues of the posterolateral vaginal corner: this reinsertion does not preserve pelvic support, which is not at risk, but ensures haemostasis of this zone. Once this haemostasis has been achieved, the operative field is dry. Just like after a simple vaginal hysterectomy, vaginal closure is limited to an overcast stitch taking hold of vaginal sections from the left to the right (*figure 10.29*).

The operative specimen is just (if not more) radical as an operative specimen as after abdominal hysterectomy (*figure*

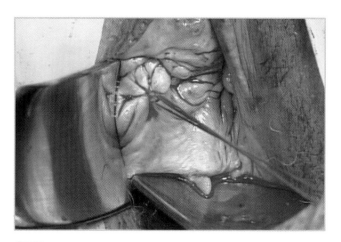

10.29 Vaginal closure.

10.30). The side effects of the operation often include transitory urinary retention. Urinary fistula is possible but rare. Several urinary disfunctions may be encountered (dysuria, stress incontinence), which are frequent after any kind of radical hysterectomy.

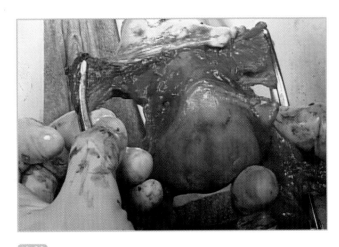

10.30 The operative specimen.

CHAPTER 11

Radical trachelectomy

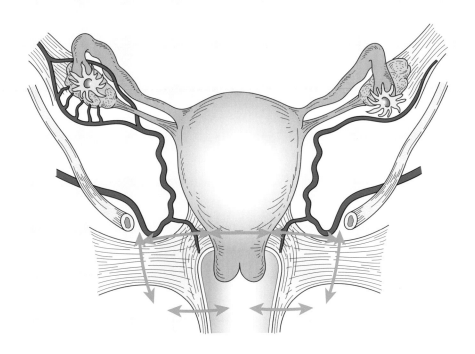

Summary sketch

Guide for the reader

Radical trachelectomy (the Dargent operation) is the prototype of the modern cancerologic operation: it provides the proof that radical cancer surgery performed via a vaginal approach must not be forgotten; adapted for small cervical tumours found during routine examination, this operation preserves a young women's capacity for motherhood, and does not produce any other scar than that resulting from pelvic lymph node dissection.

Trachelectomy is the ablation of the uterine cervix. If the remaining cervix presents a benign pathology it can be treated by simple trachelectomy, which is a technique resembling simple vaginal hysterectomy in its initial and final stages, the difference being that no extra stage is required for the uterine blood vessels and upper pedicles. If the remaining cervix is a carrier of malignant pathology, it can be treated by an operation analogous to the Schauta operation, with the same differences applicable.

Here, we will describe radical trachelectomy. It is designed to conserve the uterine body and thus the fertility in young women with cervical cancers that wish to maintain their possibility of pregnancy.

It is a proximal-type radical intervention performed by a vaginal approach, and preceded by laparoscopy performed purely for lymph node dissection. Developed by Dargent, this operation permits radical ablation of the cervix and vaginal vault (figure 11.2), while preserving the endocervix's upper part, the uterine body and the adnexae, then re-establishes the isthmo-vaginal continuity. Possibility of subsequent pregnancy can thus be preserved in cases of early cervical cancers. This intervention is, therefore, solely performed on young women with a wish for future pregnancies. It is also limited to tumours that are small (less than 20 mm) and completely exocervical, that is to say, if a sufficient tumour margin can be obtained by sectioning the upper endocervix. It should only be carried out in cases where there is no dissemination to the lymph nodes, in which case concomitant radiochemotherapy would have to be performed.

The general strategy, similar in enlarged trachelectomy and enlarged hysterectomy, is:

– Incise the vagina at the adequate height in order to obtain an adequate vaginal cuff;

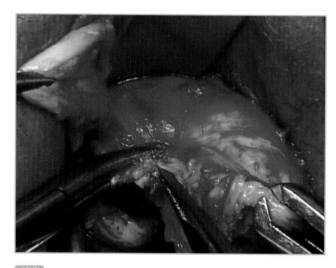

11.3 Positioning the forceps on the cervico-vaginal artery with conservation of the uterine artery. The cardinal ligament has previously been sectioned.

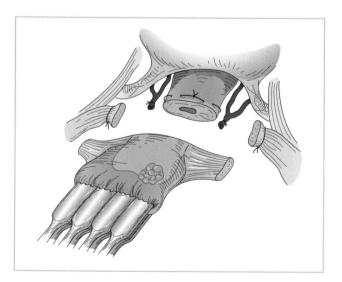

11.4 The cervico-vaginal artery has been sectioned (indicated by the dissection forceps), the conserved uterine artery is visible above the forceps.

Results obtained by radical trachelectomy

Goal of this intervention is to both treat cancer and conserve fertility. Results must, therefore, be viewed with these two factors in mind.

A Canadian controlled case study has shown that survival of patients having received conservative treatment (32 cases) is 95 % as compared to 100 % in a control group of 556 patients. Parametrial relapse was observed in only one patient with 1A2 adenocarcinoma.

Pregnancies were recorded in 19 to 37 % of cases, depending on the groups.

11.2 Principle of radical trachelectomy.

– Open the paravesical and pararectal fossae.

– Identify and dissect the ureter;

– Grip, cut and link the paracervices. Only the consecutive stages that are specific for trachelectomy will be described.

During radical trachelectomy, the uterine artery is not tied, but merely its cervical branch. The cervix is removed, then reconstituted. One identifies the uterine artery's loop, which will be preserved. After sectioning the paracervices directly below the ureter, a forceps is placed perpendicular to the cervical axis, at the height of the uterine isthmus and under the uterine artery's loop (figures 11.3 and 11.4). When this has been performed on both sides, the cervix is sectioned about 8 to 10 mm below the isthmus (figure 11.5). The cervicectomy specimen, broadened at the vaginal collar and at the region proximal to the paracervices, is now removed. At the level of the isthmus one places a permanent preventive cerclage on the uterine cervix (a calibre 8 non-resorbable thread, set around the isthmus' periphery and knotted on the posterior median line). The cervical section is closed by four Sturmdorf stiches placed on each of the cardinal points. Surrounding the cervical orifice, a crown of about 5 mm radius is left (figures 11.6 and 11.7). It is essential to avoid the vagina's invagination inside the endocervix, so as to allow subsequent colposcopic monitoring of the section's two edges, vaginal and endocervical.

Specific complications encountered during trachelectomy

Cervical stenosis is possible, provoking menstrual retention or simply difficulties in monitoring the cervix. Cervical sterility, caused by reduced mid-cycle mucus production, can occur: this is why 5 mm of endocervix are kept during the operation. Uterine relapse is possible, but has rarely been observed. Obstetrical complications include spontaneous abortion or extreme premature delivery, which are due to the loss of egg protection by the cervical canal. Prevention consists of the closing the cervical orifice. Finally, Caesarean is mandatory, due to the presence of a permanent cerclage.

An extemporaneous examination of the edge of the upper cervical section must confirm that this is intact. If this is not the case, the operation is immediately completed by hysterectomy. The patient was previously be notified of this possible outcome.

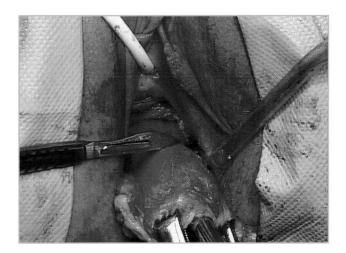

11.5   Sectioning the uterine cervix.

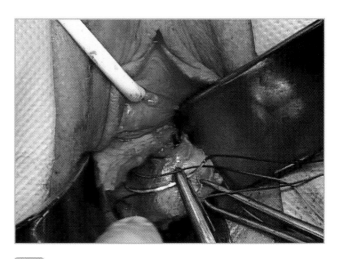

11.6   Sturmdorf stitch.

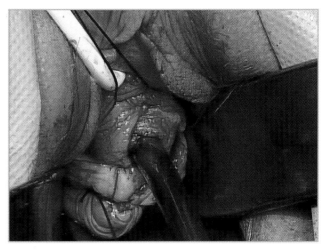

11.7   Cervix reconstituted by two Sturmdorf stiches. A bougie is placed inside the endocervix.

CHAPTER 12

Colpectomy

Guide to the reader

Colpectomy (vaginal exeresis) is paradoxically a rarity in vaginal surgery, if one does not count resection of excess tissue during surgery of a prolapse. Thus, the present chapter discusses very particular cases.

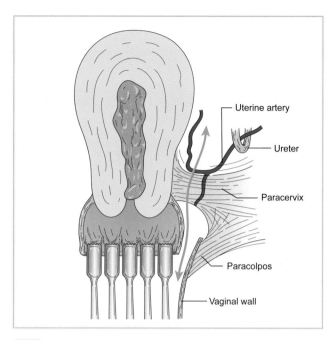

12.1 Simple complete hysterectomy with colpectomy: combination of simple colpectomy (cf. infra) and simple hysterectomy.

COLPECTOMY IN CONNECTION WITH TREATMENT OF AN ENDOMETRIOTIC CANCER

Stage IIA endometriotic cancers can be treated by extrafascial simple complete hysterectomy with colpectomy. In such cases, colpectomy is taken up after the initial stages of a Schanta operation: fashioning the cuff following the vaginal incision, opening the Douglas' pouch and vesicouterine space. One must then remove the adjacent tissue from the four vaginal fornices. The tissue in the front and the back can be removed without haemostasis, while remaining in contact with the vagina. Laterally, progressive haemostasis (electric or using forceps) are necessary, while remaining in contact with the vagina's far wall. A simple complete hysterectomy can now be commenced. This procedure will be extrafascial, since the cardinal ligaments will be treated a few millimetres from their insertion. There will be no risk to the ureter if the bladder pillar is pushed out of the way by a retractor placed within the vesicouterine septum, as required for simple complete hysterectomy (*figure 12.1*).

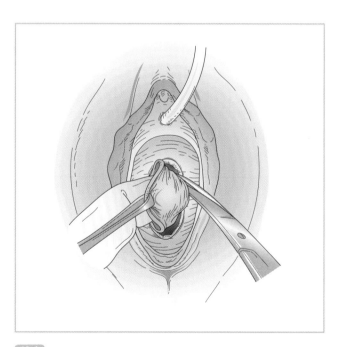

12.2 Vaginal exeresis by detachment of its deep side.

RADICAL COLPECTOMY BY VAGINAL APPROACH

During such an operation the vaginal section is performed lower down than during the Schauta operation, further away from the lesion. As a result, the cuff will be much larger.

Several variations can be described, all of which treat very specific problems.

An externalised prolapse resulting from a vaginal cancer is an indication for selection of a vaginal approach. The major points of both techniques are combined by performing a generous anterior and posterior detachment, widely opening the paravisceral fossae – easy in case of a prolapse – and vesicouterine separation. In a prolapsed or even externalised pillar of the bladder, the ureter is palpated and dissected. The distended paracervices and paracolpos are now gripped more or less laterally, according to the tumour margin required, with the ureter under direct surveillance.

Women with cancer of the middle third of the vagina that desire pregnancy represent the rare cases were radical vaginal colpectomy with uterine conservation followed by vaginal replacement with a sigmoidal graft is indicated. The procedure is completed by utero-graft anastomosis and vestibulo-graft anastomosis performed via a vaginal approach after abdominal resection of the sigmoidal graft.

COMPLETE OR SIMPLE SUBTOTAL COLPECTOMY

This concerns extended *in situ* carcinomas, often observed following hysterectomy due to cancer or precancerous lesions. In the absence of a previous hysterectomy, the entirety of the surgical intervention is concerned. However, it can be followed by a simple complete hysterectomy or even by a simple trachelectomy with uterovaginal reconstruction.

Prerequisite for a vaginal approach is complete visibility of the vaginal fundus and a certain degree of pelvic looseness, which permits close dissection without any risk to the ureter. The lower vaginal incision is located according to the lower extension of the lesions. Starting at the circular incision that cuts through the thickness of the vagina, the separation of the wall is continued by dissecting its far side, as described for a prolapse (*figure 12.2*). The dissection is very easy, except at the level of the ureter and anal canal, the fascias of which are interconnected with the vaginal fascia, and, following hysterectomy, at the level of the vaginal fundus, where the fossae of vaginal tissue have to be neatly excised. Following hysterectomy, the bladder is usually alonf side to the vaginal fundus, which it can even surpass. During abdominal surgery, this obstacle is overcome by a delicate dissection, starting with a peritoneal incision at the posterior side of the vaginal fundus. During a vaginal approach, the difficulty is often eliminated by dissecting the bladder from the intact vesicovaginal space, thus providing easiser initial cleavage, permitting better orientation.

The procedure begins by defining the lower limits of the exeresis zone with a Lugol test. The incision line is gripped with forceps, forming a circular fold into which a haemostatic liquid is infiltrated (*figure 12.3*). The fold is first incised at the front, then at the back (*figure 12.4*).

Next, one deals with the supravaginal wall. It is identified in the same manner as at the beginning of radical hysterectomy. The lower the vaginal incision, the higher up the supravaginal septum will appear to be and the more difficult to overcome

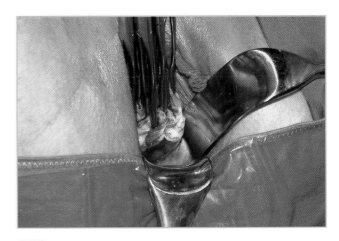
12.4 Posterior incision on the Lugol-positive zone.

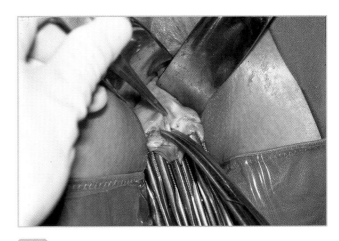
12.5 Manipulation of the supravaginal wall.

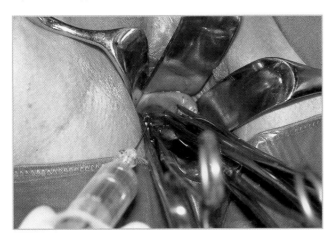
12.3 The vagina has been wiped with Lugol. Infiltration is carried out into the invagination created by the forceps.

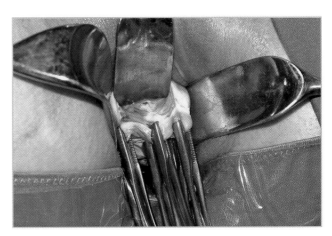
12.6 Retractor in the vesiovaginal septum.

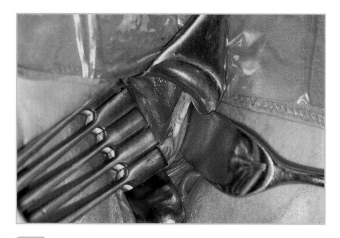

12.7 The vagina's posterior side separated from the rectum. One can begin with the right lateral incision.

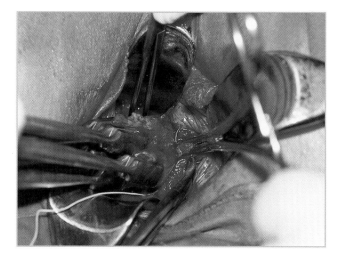

12.9 Haemostasis of the left paracolpos.

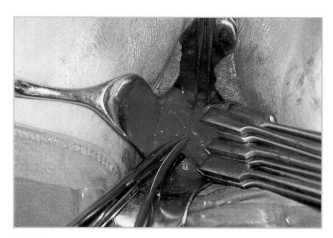

12.8 The hold on the left paracolpos.

(*figure 12.5*). The correct path lies, as usual, on the median line, half-way between the incision's edges.

This leads to the opening of the vesicovaginal septum (*figure 12.6*) into which a retractor can be placed. Only upon reaching the peritoneal pouch can one definitely be sure that the bladder has been displaced out of the way. At the back, the rectovaginal septum is reached by liberating the vagina's deep side (*figure 12.7*).

Laterally, the incision is more delicate. It is made easier by applying traction to the Chroback forceps closing the vaginal cavity (*figure 12.7*). Vaginal detachment allows to encounter, grasp (*figure 12.8*) and verify the condition of (*figure 12.9*) the paracolpos before terminating the procedure. If one remains in touch with the vagina's far side, the ureter is not at risk.

Following exeresis of the operative specimen, the vaginal incision can be closed transversally if reconstruction is not necessary. However, vaginal reconstruction can be envisaged in all cases. This will be done with a cutaneous graft, or a myocutaneous flap, or even better, a sigmoidal transplant carried out by an abdominal approach or coeliosurgery.

PARTIAL COLPECTOMY

Following its colposcopic identification, the lesion, together with a safety margin of 1 cm, is removed by localised excision via the vaginal route. The deep side of the vaginal wall is dissected in the presence or absence of haemostatic infiltrations. The suture will be transversal, bringing together the incisions upper and lower edges, rather than its lateral edges, in order to avoid stenosis. These edges must be broadly detached on their deep side in the total periphery of the operative incisions.

However, bringing together the incisions edges is difficult, and one often has to turn to the use of heterotopic tissue. In this case, anything is possible (flap from a lateral transposition, fasciocutaneous flap, myocutaneous flap). These methods remain outside the scope of the present textbook. Where the loss of substance is low to medium (up to 3 to 4 cm in diameter), the easiest method resulting in the lowest extent of scaring is the transposition of a flap, namely the Martius technique using a bulbocavernous flap with labial fat pad. The large lip's fibrous and lipid content is vascularised by both the external pudendal artery on the ventral side and the internal pudendal artery on the dorsal side: this can be used for interposition with an anterior or, more frequently, a posterior pedicle. In the latter case, it is associated with a labial fat pad that has been taken from the large lip's anterior side (*figures 12.10 and 12.11*). The supporting pedicle is reached by a vertical cutaneous incision performed on the crest of the labia. The subcutaneous cellular tissue is detached on either side of the incision, thus separating the large lip's contents. This is pedicled, and the labial tissue's ventral pole cut after haemostasis, allowing generous mobilisation of the flap.

A tunnel is created between the vaginal operative site and the excision site in order to bring the labial fat pad towards the region suffering a loss of substance where it is then sutured. The periphery of the labial fat pad is sutured to the labial tissue in order to avoid its avulsion during its passage through the tunnel linking the two operative fields. The donor site is closed over a filiform drainage or lamina. This technique can be applied bilaterally so as to obtain two islets; the only drawback of such an approach is the pilosity.

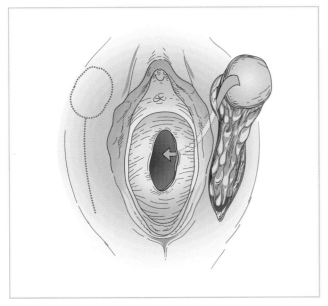

12.10   Martius' graft with labial fat pad.
Vaginal defect following partial colpectomy.
Indicated on the left: Incision of the large lip and a sketch of the pad.
Indicated on the right: Removal of the flap, which is pedicled onto the lower external pudendal blood vessels.

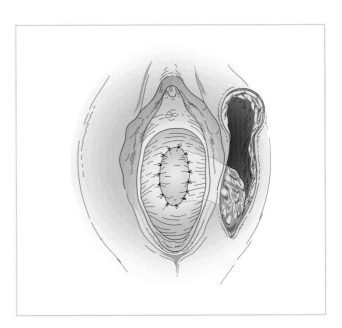

12.11   Martius' graft with labial fat pad.
The pad is transplanted towards the defect via a tunnel linking the large lip to the vaginal cavity.

Prolapse

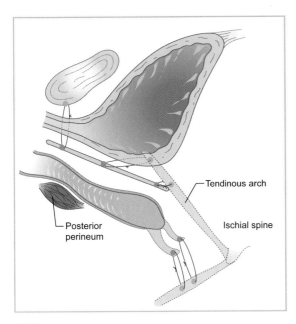

PART 5

1 Prolapse treatment via a vaginal approach: "Plastron", Richter and myorraphy.

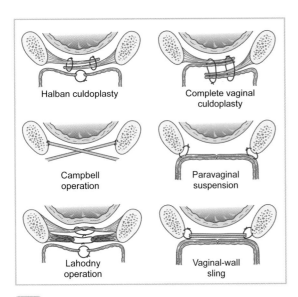

2 Different cystocele treatments.

Classic techniques (*figure 1*)

Vaginal colpohysterectomy.
"Plastron" in case of a large cystocele.
Campbell operation.
Douglassectomy in case of elytrocele.
Richter operation: sacrospinous suspension.
Myorrhaphy of the levator muscles.
If necessary, urinary intervention.

Techniques for curing genital prolapses

We will not repeat in detail the indications for surgical prolapse treatment. Since this is an operation aimed at improving comfort, such interventions should not be performed unless dysfunction is related to the volume of externalised prolapse, or unless the prolapse is causing urinary or ano-rectal problems. A careful and exhaustive case review must be performed before deciding on a surgical intervention. The advantages and disadvantages must be discussed in detail with the patient in order to obtain her informed consent.

To this end, the anatomic and functional benefits must be clearly separated. The anatomic benefit of the operation is all the more important if the patient presents a bothersome and voluminous exteriorisation. However, urinary and digestive dysfunction are often tolerated less well than progressive swelling, and complications or after-effects of the operation are not easily accepted if the patient had not been correctly informed. The preoperative case review is, therefore, essential and should include both the clinical classification stage of the genital prolapse, as well as a qualitative and quantitative evaluation of concomitant symptoms. Dysfunction, such as urinary incontinence, should be evaluated and quantified objectively (pad test). A precise evaluation includes the degree of urinary and ano-rectal symptoms, as well as their effects on the patient's quality of life. Finally, the patient must be fully informed on the advantages, disadvantages and possible after-effects the operation can bring to their sexuality. If a patient is hesitant, she must be fully informed about any benefits and drawbacks of medical or surgical treatment and be given ample time to think it over before making up her mind.

Indications are the following:

– genital prolapse objectively determined;
– the case having been subject to a complete review with regard to urinary and ano-rectal functioning;
– a situation affecting the patient's quality of life and/or sexuality;
– the patient having been informed about the benefits and drawbacks brought about by surgical intervention;
– the patient accepting the risks of failure and eventual secondary after-effects;
– the operation is most frequently performed on patients not desiring subsequent pregnancy.

We will describe in this next part of the book some of the procedures, and different operative stages that are often associated in routine practice. The focus will always be on completely curing a prolapse affecting the three levels of the statics of the pelvis, the development of which will be closely followed. In our team, this technique more often than not associates colpohysterectomy, a vaginal-wall sling for curing cystocele and the crossing of the subsymphyseal uterosacral ligaments according to Campbell's technique before completing the intervention by suspending the vaginal vault according to Richter and performing a myorrhaphy of the levator muscles.

We will report on a few of the techniques that can be applied for curing a cystocele. Among the different possible technique, we will mention (figure 1): the Halban culdoplasty or complete vaginal culdoplasty; the Lahodny intervention, the Campbell technique, as well as techniques for paravaginal suspension, and the vaginal-wall sling (referred to in this work as the "plastron" technique). Only the latter three, which we perform on a regular basis, will be discussed in more detail.

Of course, we will subsequently discuss techniques for treating genital prolapse with uterine conservation, such as the Richardson and Manchester techniques (figure 3). We will present the techniques for paravaginal suspension that have inspired the vaginal-wall sling approach, as well as perineal reconstruction according to Musset, which is a beautiful intervention that is only rarely necessary nowadays.

We have followed our principle put forward at the beginning of this textbook that we will merely discuss those techniques that we regularly perform ourselves. The techniques for colporrhaphy with vaginal resection, which we do not perform anymore, have thus not been included (though they are still very much present in operating rooms!). Likewise, those techniques that are widely found in surgical atlases, but for which we do not have any experience, will not be described. These include treatment urinary incontinence according to Marion-Kelly, bursa of the prerectal or prevesical fascia, high prerectal myorrhaphy, and subvesical ventral myorrhaphy.

The exact role of any one of these various techniques has not been determined in a rational manner. The best technique for treatment of a prolapse by abdominal or vaginal approach remains the subject of heated discussions, with disputes between different schools; the surgeon's personal convictions often provides the sole determining factor for the choice of a given technique. Insufficient evaluation, a nearly complete absence of randomised studies and, finally, rapid evolution of surgical techniques partially explain this situation. It also explains the ephemeral character of such chapters describing techniques that will surely be modified or even be commented with pity in only a few years' time...

This is nevertheless the general rule of the exercise, and we will not claim to be exempt. We will discuss some surgical techniques that have not yet been evaluated, but appear to be promising or thought provoking; or that use interesting materials – particularly prolene prostheses – or approach routes (figure 4).

Finally, this introduction will not be complete without mentioning preoperative infiltrations that we perform on a routine basis. If, in the case of vaginal hysterectomy, the infiltration is useful to improve vision by reducing minor bleedings, it finds its full justification during genital prolapse surgery. In this intervention that involves extended dissection a correctly administered infiltration prepares the dissection spaces, thus playing the role of aqua-dissection described for laparoscopic surgery. The infiltration must be applied neither too superficially nor too deeply in the vaginal wall, but inside the dissection space itself. Infiltration in a wrong plane could lead to an incorrect dissection plane, not mentioning the risk of an intravascular injection. After obtaining the anaesthetist's consent, the injection mixture is prepared with three adrenaline-containing Xylocaïne vials diluted, as required, in three to nine vials of physiological serum.

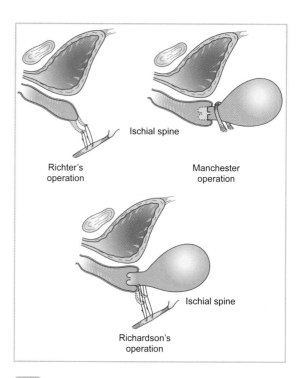

3 Different techniques to suspend the vaginal cuff.

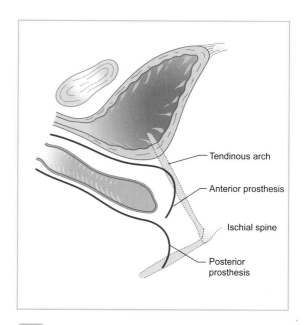

4 Curing a prolapse by prosthesis.

CHAPTER 13

Vaginal colpohysterectomy

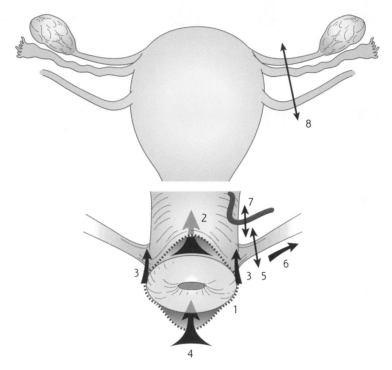

13.1   *Summary sketch.*
1. Pericervical incision. 2. Vesicovaginal dissection and opening of the anterior pouch. 3. Pericervical dissection. 4. Dissection and opening the Douglas' pouch. 5. Sectioning the uterosacral ligaments. 6. Dissection of the uterosacral ligaments in cases of associated Campbell's operation. 7. Uterine ligature and sectioning. 8. Ligature and sectioning of the utero-ovarian and round ligaments.

Guide to the reader

1. Description of the operative stages that can precede hysterectomy during treatment of prolapse.
2. Detailed description of the different techniques in relation to simple hysterectomy prior to sectioning the uterine arteries.
3. Defining the chronology of events by distinguishing between dissection and sectioning.
4. Identifying the operative stages where technical difficulties could be encountered, and possible solutions.

Even if vaginal hysterectomy is not indispensable before treatment of a genital prolapse by a vaginal approach, it is, nevertheless, often performed in association with the latter intervention; in aged women, where conservation is but rarely required, the technique is easy and rapidly performed, and, since screening for and treatment of endometriotic pathologies becomes more difficult, its association is also of a preventive nature. Furthermore, secondary hysterectomy will prove difficult and dangerous to carry out by a vaginal approach following (or not) direct suspension of the organ. Uterine conservation renders efficient action via a vaginal approach more difficult. This is due to the posterior orientation of the suspension to the uterosacral ligaments following Richardson's technique for suspension to the sacrospinous ligaments, which result in uterine tipping and bending of the uterine cervix. Even though it is technically simple, conservation of the uterine cervix by subtotal vaginal hysterectomy is not a frequently used method.

TECHNICAL PRINCIPLES

Vaginal infiltration prepares the dissections.
The pericervical dissections are similar to those during radical colpohysterectomy according to Schauta.
In the case of cervical elongation, several ligature stages of the suspending ligaments are sometimes necessary.
The operative stages are similar to those of simple hysterectomy, apart from those for treating cervical elongation, where applicable.

Technically, the operation is very similar to vaginal hysterectomy carried out in the absence of a genital prolapse. The differences are in part due to uterine externalisation, facilitating certain operative stages, and in part due to the frequently observed cervical elongation, which renders these same stages more delicate. It also differs from the so-called simple hysterectomy since associated anterior and posterior suspensions must be anticipated. Thus, the frequent use of uterosacral ligaments requires an extended dissection before sectioning the uterine

cervix at its far end. The presence of elytrocele requires dissection and resection of the sac prior to peritonisation. This peritonisation is not indispensable in the absence of treatment for a prolapse, but becomes necessary in connection to a suspension according to Richter in order to avoid contact between the dissected pararectal fossae and the small intestines. Finally, in cases of action for suspension or vesical support one must prepare the anterior incision even before performing the pericervical incision, since its realisation and visualisation is easier as long as the cervix can still be used for orientation and for applying traction.

DESCRIPTION

Here we will describe a colpohysterectomy performed during a complete surgical treatment of genital prolapse, including treatment of cystocele by the plastron technique and suspension of the uterosacral ligaments according to Campbell, followed by suspension of the vaginal cuff according to Richter.

Infiltration

For colpohysterectomy, this infiltration is performed pericervically, inside the anterior and posterior dissection spaces, and laterally in front of the suspending ligaments. The required volume varies between 40 to 50 cm^3. It might be necessary to perform an associated infiltration related with to the associated actions of suspension. Ideally, not more than three adrenaline-containing Xylocaïne vials should be used in total; the dilution will, therefore, be adapted to the total infiltration volume according to the total number of actions to be performed.

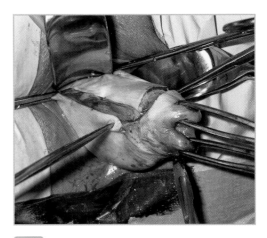

13.2 View of the pericervical incision and the incision.

Performing the anterior incision

In case of the plastron technique (cf. chapter 16), the incision is performed prior to pericervical incision (figure 13.2). In case of a "T"-incision, one commences with the median anterior incision. This incision is carried out while exposing the incision path with the help of Kocher forceps. The incision is performed inbetween the forceps, the edges are then grasped using Allis' forceps and the incision is continued in the location where the Kocher forceps had previously been positioned.

Pericervical incision

The pericervical incision (figure 13.2) is performed with a cold scalpel by uniformly incising the vagina. This is in contrast to the pericervical incision performed at the beginning of a vaginal hysterectomy carried out in the case of benign pathology in the absence of a prolapse. In fact, it is most often necessary to do a pericervical vaginal dissection that could not be performed in case of superficial incisions on the incision's lateral regions. Once the incision has been performed, the Allis' forceps are positioned its edges.

Vesicovaginal dissection

Prior to carrying out the hysterectomy itself, it is advisable to perform a vesical dissection in order to prepare the treatment of cystocele. This is easier before hysterectomy, when the cervix is still in place, thus allowing firm traction, while at the same time being favourable for the subsequent uterovesical dissection. This dissection is initiated with a cold scalpel by distancing the Allis' forceps from each other, which exposes the operative field. The bladder is grasped with a toothless forceps and the space that is thereby opened is incised. The dissection is continued with the finger or a compress in order to push back the bladder. One does not go so far as to open the paravesical trenches so as not to augment the duration of bleeding brought about by extended dissections prior to performing the suspension, that is to say prior to having completed vaginal colpohysterectomy. This stage is illustrated in the chapter discussing Campbell's procedure or the "plastron" technique and will not be discussed at this point, since it does not really form part of a hysterectomy.

Vesicouterine dissection

This is commenced by a firm anterior incision, perpendicular to the uterine cervix, leading up to the point of contact. One can now lift the bladder by applying traction with a toothless forceps and, by dissecting the space appearing on the median

line with scissors, push back the bladder with the help of a retractor. Laterally, the two pillars of the bladder become visible (figure 13.3).

Ligature-sectioning the bladder's pillars

A Jean-Louis Faure forceps is positioned on the bladder's pillars and, following sectioning and ligature using a no. 1 thread, the forceps are removed. Sectioning the two pillars opens up the uterovesical space and allows its complete dissection (figure 13.4).

Completed vesicouterine dissection

This dissection is completed by laterally pushing back the bladder on the median plane with the help of a finger or a compress. Positioning a retractor now allows the visualisation of the anterior pouch (figure 13.5).

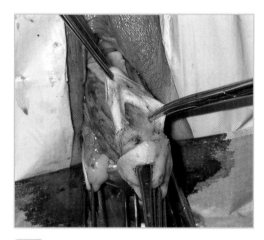

13.3 Vesicouterine dissection, pillars of the bladder.

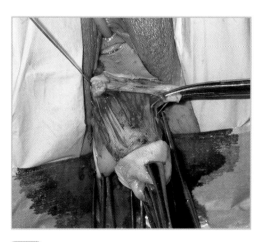

13.4 Sectioned pillars, continuation of the dissection.

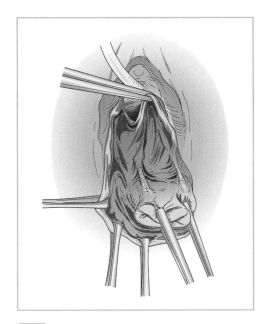

13.5 Vesicouterine dissection, anterior pouch is visible.

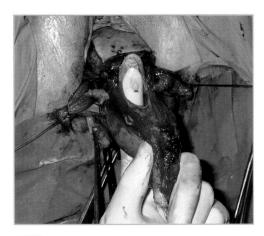

13.6 Opening the anterior pouch on the finger.

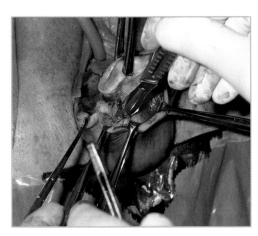

13.7 Pericervical dissection.

In case of injury to the bladder

The diagnosis must be confirmed by placing a coloured substance inside the bladder, which allows objective assessment of the bladder's wound. Suturing of the bladder's injury is performed by an overcast suture with a resorption thread. The suture's tightness is verified by again testing with the blue dye.

A urinary catheter with free drainage will be left in place for 5 to 8 days, depending on the wound's size and localisation. In case of doubt, a urological assessment will be required.

Opening the anterior pouch

The anterior peritoneal pouch can now be grasped and opened up with scissors before enlarging the incision and placing a retractor inside it. This opening is preferably performed at this stage of the intervention, since putting in place the anterior retractor allows to distance the bladder during the following operative stages (*figure 13.6*), especially during pericervical dissection, and to distance the ureters during ligature-sectioning the uterine pedicles.

The stages on the anterior area having thus been accomplished, one can now begin the posterior stages.

In case of difficulty in opening the anterior pouch

In this case it is better to perform the opening following the posterior operative stages, and after having achieved uterine rotation, as is done during hysterectomies in the absence of a prolapse (*figure 13.6*). One frequently encounters difficulties in opening the anterior or posterior peritoneal pouch in cases of cervical elongation. Following cervical dissection, one must in such cases ligature-section the suspending ligaments in order to augment uterine mobility before opening the Douglas' pouch.

Pericervical vaginal dissection

Before opening the Douglas' pouch one performs the pericervical vaginal dissection, which allows lateral mobilisation of the bladder in the front, as well as mobilisation of the uterosacral and suspending ligaments further back.

Now, tension is applied on the Allis' forceps by pulling them apart, thus permitting one to distinguish the dissection space. This dissection is also initiated with a cold scalpel before continuing with a finger (*figure 13.7*). Without contact with the vagina, this space lies halfway between the vagina and suspending ligaments, and can easily be located. The dissection is extended laterally as far as possible in order to provide a maximal length of ligament to be used during Campbell's procedure (*figure 13.8*).

Opening the Douglas' pouch

If possible, it is advantageous to open the Douglas' pouch prior to sectioning the suspending ligaments, since their sectioning, in the opposite scenario, might otherwise not be complete (*figure 13.9*). As for hysterectomies, the pouch is opened using scissors during interventions for benign lesions before enlarging the opening so as to place a Mangiagallli retractor inside it (*figure 13.10*).

Difficulties in opening the Douglas' pouch
Hypertrophic elongation of the cervix can hamper this opening, especially if the uterus turns out to be only weakly mobile or even fixed. In such cases it is sometimes necessary to perform a partial ligature-section in order to mobilise the uterus. The handling of the uterosacral ligaments will often be incomplete and will have to be repeated. One will carefully examine this, especially if one wishes to later perform an associated suspension of these ligaments below the symphysis. In such a case, the Douglas' pouch will be opened secondarily and the surgeon will check for persistent non-sectioned suspending ligaments with his index finger.

Ligature-sectioning the uterosacral and suspending ligaments

Having opened the Douglas' pouch, one will now ligature-section the uterosacral ligaments after having positioned a Jean-Louis Faure forceps. This ligature is preventively doubled and

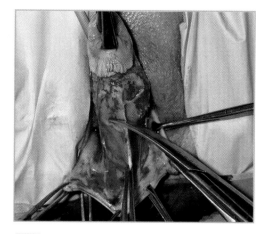

13.9 Opening the Douglas' pouch.

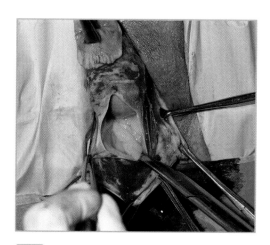

13.10 Opened Douglas' pouch.

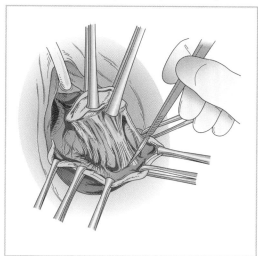

13.8 Posterior dissection, visualisation of the uterosacral ligaments.

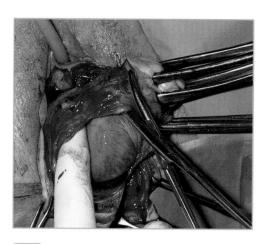

13.11 Grasping the right uterosacral ligament.

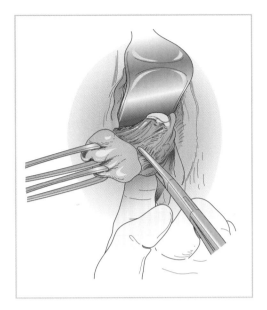

13.12 Grasping the left uterosacral ligament.

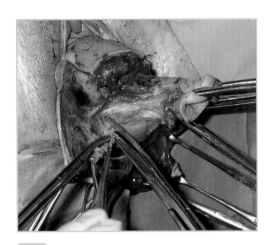

13.13 Dissecting the right uterosacral ligament.

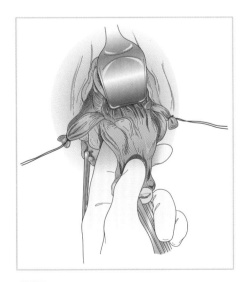

13.14 View of the right uterine pedicle.

the needled thread kept long in order to locate the ligament in relation to the Campbell's technique during the operative stage (*figure 13.11*). Contrary to the vaginal hysterectomy technique in the absence of a prolapse, using a Deschamps' needle is not helpful, since access is facilitated by the prolapse. Furthermore, in our technique, using the Deschamps' needle would results in a bringing together of the uterine artery and the sacrospinous ligament, which would not permit suspension of the uterosacral ligaments according to Campbell. This ligature is first performed on the right (*figure 13.11*) and then on the left (*figure 13.12*).

Complementary dissection of the uterosacral ligaments in case of a Campbell intervention

After having sectioned the ligament, it is desirable to have the possibility to extend its dissection – as has already been done on the vaginal side by dissecting the ligament from the parametrium – in order to allow its secondary ascent behind the symphysis. This procedure is first performed for the right then the left ligament (*figure 13.13*).

In the absence of Campbell's procedure

In such a case it is not useful to perform an extensive dissection of the uterine suspending ligaments, as these ligaments remain suspended to the angles of the vaginal incision. Numerous surgeons prefer to sagittally then transversally terminate the anterior colporrhaphy in relation to the pericervical incision, and to utilise these ligaments for a bilateral suspension to the sacrospinous ligaments.

Ligature-sectioning of the uterine arteries

Section of the suspending ligaments exposes the uterine pedicles, which can be revealed by pushing backwards with a finger (*figure 13.14*). One can now ligature-section the uterine arteries by positioning a Jean-Louis Faure forceps on

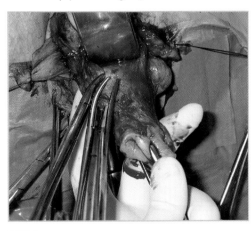

13.15 Grasping the pedicle, placing the forceps.

the visualised uterine pedicles (*figure 13.15*). The forceps is positioned at 45° to the median line, going all the way to the level of the uterus. The section is followed by a ligature with a threaded needle that is subsequently doubled.

This is preceded by a dissection of the forceps' point, which is liberated by sectioning. The pedicle is now lightly dissected by applying traction on the Jean-Louis Faure's forceps so as to facilitate its individualisation and threading (figure 13.16). These threads do not need to be kept long, as accidental traction could result in inopportune release of the suture.

If in doubt about the ureter's localisation, especially where a voluminous associated cystocele is present, it can be useful to palpate the ureter at this stage of the intervention before placing the forceps on the uterine pedicle. It is easily detected between two fingers, 1 to 2 cm above the uterine loop. Nevertheless, palpation is most efficient once the anterior and posterior pouches are open.

Posterior rotation of the uterus and verification of the adnexae

The uterus is in most cases of small volume and can easily be tipped towards the back and its floor externalised. This allows determination of the ovaries' condition. If the anterior pouch has not yet been opened, one can pass a finger behind the uterus and, while bulging it forwards with the index finger, open the pouch with scissors without any risk (*figure 13.16*). One can now place an anterior retractor.

Ligature-section of the utero-ovarian ligaments

If one wishes to perform an annexectomy, the technique is exactly as already described for simple hysterectomy, involving the round ligament's ligature-section and then opening of the broad ligament before a twofold ligature-section of the ovarian vascular pedicle. Likewise, if the patient's ovaries are to be preserved, a twofold ligature-section of the utero-ovarian pedicle will be performed (*figure 13.17*). This ligature makes use of the Heaney stitch already described in the chapter on simple vaginal hysterectomy.

Peritonisation by a purse-string closure (2/0)

With the help of a finger one can easily check for the presence of an elytrocele, which, if necessary, will be dissected as

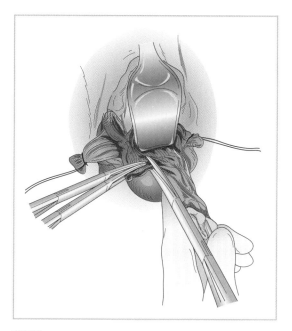

13.16 Dissection of the extremity of the right uterine pedicle's.

Checking haemostasis

At this stage of the intervention with the uterus already having been ablated, one places a gauze pad so as to push the small intestines back with the help of a large retractor. Quality of the haemostasis can systematically be verified and, if necessary, pedicles can be treated again by an "X" stitch that has been carefully performed. If in doubt, palpating the uterer is easy and can sometimes be reassuring before positioning an possible haemostasis stitch.

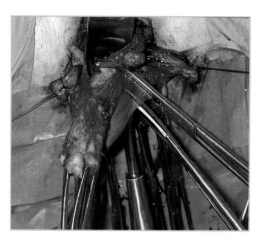

13.17 Grasping the utero-ovarian ligament.

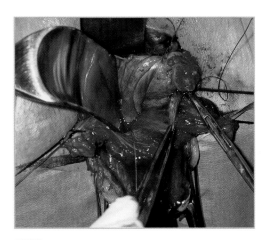

13.18 Peritonisation

Finishing anterior stage and subsequent vaginal closure

Before vaginal closure the bladder has to be suspended anteriorly. Vaginal closure can then be perform either sagittally, bringing together the utero-ovarian or round ligaments, or transversally, by leaving the uterosacral and utero-ovarian ligaments attached to the vaginal angles.

The classical sagittal closure will be preferred where a unilateral suspension has been performed according to Richter, while a transversal closure is more logical after bilateral suspension according to Richter in order to provide some space between the lateral suspensions.

Some surgeons will use the suspending ligaments to attach the vaginal vault to the sacrospinal ligaments, as previously discussed.

The vaginal colpohysterectomy stage must be completed by a quick counting of the compresses as well as a control of the haemostasis before continuing with the posterior suspension stage.

Persistent haemorrhage

If at the end of the procedure there is persistent haemorrhage:

– verify haemostasis by repositioning the retractors;

– check the pedicles and dissection spaces;

– in case of localised haemorrhage establish haemostasis;

– in case of diffuse haemorrhage of low importance in a dissection space, place a vaginal drainage gauze for 24 hours, urinary catheter with free drainage for 24 hours that is clamped during the first two hours following injection of 200 cm^3 into the bladder.

indicated in chapter 19. Following this operative stage, or in the absence of an elytrocele, the peritoneum will be closed with a purse-string formed with 2/0 resorbable thread that is passed with close stitches through the posterior peritoneum (*figure 13.18*), the right pedicles (which are sub-peritonealised), the anterior peritoneum and left pedicles, before again taking up the posterior peritoneum. Before the purse-string closure is finished, the gradual removal of the gauze is done while

We prefer to do this peritonisation, especially where the vaginal vault has been suspended according to the associated Richter technique. In fact, the small intestines are at risk of getting caught inside the pararectal fossae, even though we are not aware of any case where such a complication arose. Furthermore, in this type of operation where dissection spaces are extensive and the risk of a haematoma more elevated, it is advisable to avoid leaving the peritoneal cavity and dissection spaces in contact with each other.

verifying that (a) there is no active haemorrhage and (b) there is no protuberance of the small intestine or tube into the orifice.

CHAPTER 14

Anterior operational stages – Campbell intervention

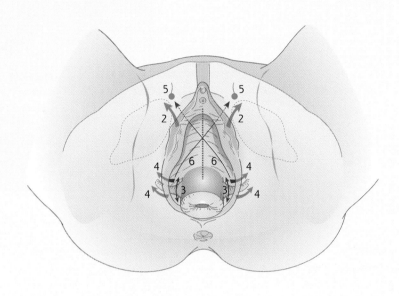

14.1 *Summary sketch.*
1. Median incision. 2. Vesicovaginal and subsymphyseal dissection. 3. Section of the uterosacral ligaments.
4. Dissection of the uterosacral ligaments. 5. Placing the points of suspension. 6. Suspending the uterosacral
ligaments.

Guide to the reader

1. Describe the indications for the Campbell intervention.
2. Define the operative stages as well as their association with other procedures during treatment of prolapse
via a vaginal approach.
3. Name the conditions required for this technique, as well as the main criteria for its success.

*C*ampbell's intervention consists of crossing the two uterosacral ligaments under the pubic symphysis. It requires the association of a vaginal colpohysterectomy and the presence of two uterosacral ligaments of good quality, a sufficient length of which is dissected to allow their ascent as far as the pubic symphysis. The main inconvenience of this intervention lies in its principle itself: ascent of the uterosacral ligaments under the pubic symphysis can result in a reduction of the vaginal diameter. This risk is even greater if the ligaments have not been sufficiently dissected and, in particular, liberated from their vaginal attachments.

INDICATION

Where a large cystocele is present, Campbell's intervention must be combined with a more specific treatment for cystocele.

SIMILAR SURGICAL INTERVENTION

Dissection of the uterosacral ligaments is similar during the Manchester intervention.

DESCRIPTION

Here we describe Campbell's procedure associated with a vaginal colpohysterectomy in a patient without a marked cystocele. The order of the actions will vary if associated with the subvesical "plastron", but, as the principal stages of this procedure will be discussed elsewhere (*cf.* chapter 16), we have decided to describe the intervention without an associated treatment for cystocele. In this case, the intervention will commence by an anterior "T"-shaped incision instead of an incision of the plastron.

Infiltration and anterior "T"-shaped incision

The infiltration is performed ounding to the line of incision and inside the lateral vesicovaginal detachment spaces.

It is guided by two Kocher forceps marking the beginning and end of the anterior incision. Of course, this infiltration is related to a preparative pericervical infiltration for vaginal colpohysterectomy. The pericervical incision is referred to as a "T"-shaped incision, due to its median anterior vaginal extension that starts more or less at the uterovesical junction, identifiable by the distension of the urinary probe, and ends at the pericervical incision. Following this firm incision, the Allis' forceps are put into place (*figure 14.2*).

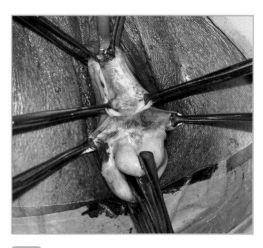

14.2 T"-shaped incision and vesicovaginal dissection.

Vesiaginal dissection

This dissection is classic and performed as described in chapter 22 that deals with the Manchester intervention. The lateral dissection does not include a complete opening of the paravesical fossae, since this is not required for subsymphyseal suspension. This dissection must liberate the bladder's anterior side in order to permit the lifting of the uterosacral ligaments under the bladder, usually all the way to the vaginal pouch.

Subsymphyseal dissection

The subsymphyseal dissection liberates the anterior side of the pubic symphysis, and notably its subsymphyseal part by starting into Retzius' space in order to obtain the sufficient room to carry out the subsymphyseal stiches.

Vaginal colpohysterectomy

We will merely discuss two operative stages that present some particularities:
– the uterosacral ligaments' section must be detailed, since it requires sectioning as near as possible to the uterine contact in order to maintain a maximum length for the uterosacral ligaments;

– the uterosacral ligaments' dissection (*figure 14.3*) is essential for the same reason, and also for liberating them from the vesical floor and the ureters, and laterally from the uterine arteries and the vagina, so that their ascent during suspension does not result in a vaginal narrowing, vesical rotation, or even traction on the uterine pedicles or a bending of the ureters.

Positioning the suspension thread

Placing these two stitches is described in conjunction with the "plastron" technique (*cf.* chapter 16).

The passage of the first stitch on the patient's left side is technically easier. Having moved the vaginal pouch out of the way with the help of the Allis' forceps, the needle is presented by the needle-holder, perpendicular to the lower part of the pubic rami (*figure 14.1*). The needle grazes along the osseous branch for 1 to 2 cm before being grasped with an empty needle-holder. One must make sure that the needle is not transfixing at the vaginal level. If one encounters difficulties in placing this stitch, one can place the Allis' forceps at the level of the vaginal pouch in order to facilitate its location. A right-handed surgeon will pass the needle from front to back for the left stitch, and from back to front for the right stitch, the risk of transfixion being more elevated on the right side. Once the stitch has been placed, its stability must be tested by applying firm traction.

Suspending the uterosacral ligaments

Having placed the suspension stitches, the dissected uterosacral ligaments must merely be taken up by the suspension thread. The ligaments' length is compared and the shorter one chosen for the first suspension. The longer one can then easily pass over the first. The ligaments are crossed below the pubic symphysis. The right ligament is always suspended with the left thread and vice versa; only the order of suspension remains to be determined. The non-resorbable suspension thread is taken up with the needle-holder and passed twice through the ligament. The first passage will transfix the ligament behind the uterosacral ligament's ligature, while the second passage will be supported by this ligature. The stability is tested before performing the same suspension procedure contralaterally (*figure 14.5*).

Closing the anterior vaginal wall

The intervention can be finished with a subvesical purse-string sutures, which we do not perform, or another technique for the treatment of a cystocele. Once the anterior procedure

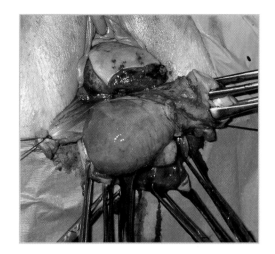

14.3 The right uterosacral ligament has been ligatured, sectioned and dissected.

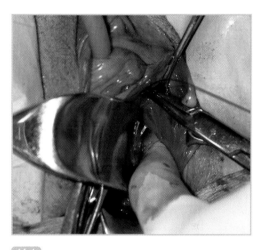

14.4 Passing the needle for retrosymphyseal suspension.

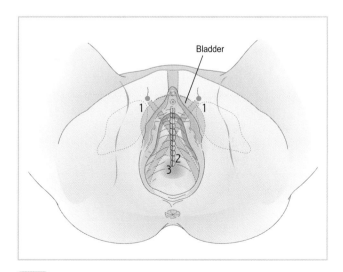

14.5 Final result of the surgical intervention.
1. Crossed uterosacral ligaments in retrosymphyseal suspension.
2. Anterior colporraphy. 3. Vaginal vault.

has been completed, the compresses counted and haemostasis controlled, the anterior colpotomy will be closed with a continuous overcast suture.

In case of association with "plastron" procedure
The main operative stages are as follows:
– infiltration, plastron incision, vesicovaginal dissection;
– vaginal colpohysterectomy with dissection of the uterosacral ligaments, which are kept free;
– opening the paravesical fossae and dissection of the pelvic fascia's tendinous arches;
– suspension of the plastron, the subsymphyseal suspension thread is maintained for suspension of the uterosacral ligaments;
– crossing the uterosacral ligaments in retrosymphyseal suspension;
– closing the anterior colpotomy.

CHAPTER 15

Anterior operative stages – Paravaginal suspension to the tendinous arches of the pelvic fascia

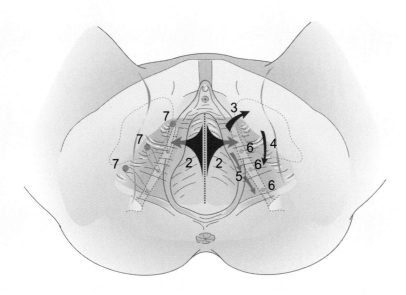

15.1 *Summary sketch.*
1. Median incision. 2. Vesicovaginal incision and beginning of the opening of the paravesical fossae.
3. Opening the paravesical fossa. 4. Enlarging the fossa with a finger. 5. Dissection – palpating the
tendinous arch. 6. Placing the three suspension points for the tendinous arches. 7. Suspending the lateral vaginal pouch.

Guide to the reader

1. Describe the technique for vesical dissection and opening of the paravesical fossae.
2. Anatomically locate the tendinous arches of the pelvic fascia.
3. Detail the procedure for placing the suspension threads.
4. Identify the anatomical structures at risk of lesion during the course of this procedure, the prevention of this
   risk and treatment of such complications.

*S*urgical treatment of cystocele by paravaginal
suspension has been described by Baden and
Walker. The principle of this intervention is to
link the anterior vaginal pouch to the pelvic
fascia's tendinous arches by placing suspension
points between these elements. This technique
has brought a new therapeutic approach to
cystocele treatment, which until then was
based on anterior colpectomy techniques, or,
in the best of cases, on the attachment of the
vesical floor to Halban's fascia by supports, or
to the prevesical tissues which do not have the
appropriate qualities for suspension. It is neither
useful nor desirable to perform vaginal resection
with this technique, and its main advantage
compared to the "plastron" method is that it
can be carried out even without an excess of
vaginal tissue. However, putting the vaginal
pouches into place results in their marked ascent,
as well as their lateral repositioning, which
can result in difficulties during closure. On the
other hand, this lateral strengthening is efficient
for the treatment of lateral cystoceles, but will
not prevent a subsequent median cystocele.
Another advantage of this technique is that
posterior vaginal suspension, by suspension to
the sacrospinous ligaments, is not necessary. In
fact, direct suspension of the vaginal pouches can
theoretically permit this to be done alone (even
though an isolated cystocele may rarely occur), or
even to be carried out with uterine conservation.

INDICATION

The intervention is indicated for the treatment of moderate
cystoceles via a vaginal approach, regardless of the patient's
age.

RELATED TECHNIQUES

This technique can be compared to:
– cystocele treatment by the "plastron" technique, for its the
suspension to the tendinous arches;

– culdoplasty for vesical dissection, for the vesical dissection
and lateral fixation of the vaginal pouches;
– Campbell's procedure, for the steps of incision and vesical
dissection.

DESCRIPTION

We will quickly describe the procedure, which we do not
perform in this way. It essentially corresponds to the stages
following the incision and describes the vesical dissection illustrated in chapter 14 on Campbell's procedure, followed by the
passing of threads inside the tendinous arches as described for
the "plastron" intervention stages (chapter 16). The main difference consists of the direct suspension of the vaginal pouches
to the pelvic fascia's tendinous arches. In our experience, its
main application lies in the creation of a prosthetic "plastron"
as indicated in chapter 23, which discusses novel techniques
that are currently being evaluated. The operative stages will be
described to a minimum at this point, since they are already
discussed elsewhere in this manual.

Anterior vaginal incision

(Cf. Campbell's procedure, chapter 14)
As usual, we will commence by placing Kocher forceps and
performing the vaginal infiltration into the dissection plane.
The median incision is followed by the positioning of the Allis'
forceps.

Dissection of the bladder

(Cf. Campbell's procedure, chapter 14)
Having separated the Allis' forceps from each other and
applied traction to them, the bladder is dissected as far as the
lateral vaginal pouches.

Opening the paravesical spaces

(Cf. Plastron technique, chapter 16)
The paravesical fossae are now dissected so as to place a
retractor inside that will protect the bladder (*figure 15.2*).

Dissection of the tendinous arches

(Cf. Plastron technique, chapter 16)
The dissection is usually performed with a finger and preceded by a palpation for the location of the tendinous arches.
It liberates the two most fleshy centimetres of the tendinous
arch's pre-obturator portion.

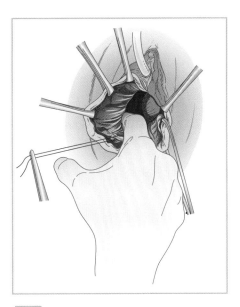

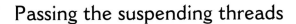 Opening the paravesical spaces.

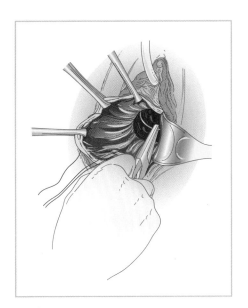 Three threads have been placed on the right, the bladder is held back with a retractor.

Passing the suspending threads

(*Cf.* "Plastron" technique, chapter 16)

Once dissected, the pelvic fascia's tendinous arches are taken up with two non-resorbable threads on each side. Placing the threads is most frequently done blindly, with the left index finger of a right-handed surgeon guiding the needle (*figure 15.3*).

Suspension of the vaginal pouches

These same non-resorbable suspension threads will be passed through the vagina's thickness without transfixing the vaginal pouches. As in all techniques for vaginal suspension without vaginal strip, this operative stage depends on the vaginal tissue's quality and, particularly, on its thickness. Passing the threads will be more difficult and risks transfixation if the vaginal tissue is atrophic; this could result in a vaginal granuloma that might require subsequent section of the suspending thread. Furthermore, the vaginal hold is more fragile in such a case: the thread will have to be passed several times through the vaginal thickness, thus distributing the suspension over all of the lateral pouch (*figure 15.4*).

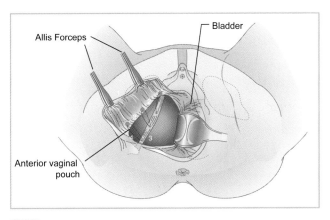

15.4 Suspension of the vaginal pouches.
1. Anterior vaginal wall lifted with Allis' forceps. 2. Identification of the lateral vaginal pouch. 3. Tendinous arch with suspending threads put into place. 4. Suspension of the vaginal pouch by non-transfixing stitches.

Closing the anterior vaginal wall

After having counted the compresses, the anterior vaginal wall is closed with a crossed overcasting suture and without vaginal resection, in order to avoid closing under tension (*figure 15.5*).

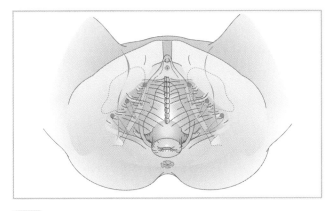

15.5 Final view.

CHAPTER 16

Anterior operational stages – the "Plastron" technique

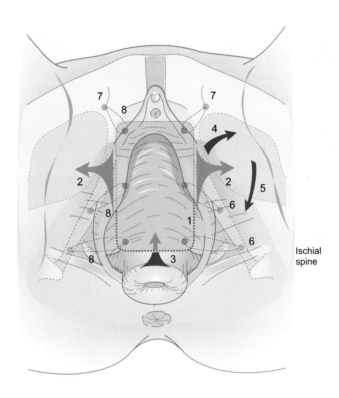

16.1 *Summary sketch.*
1. Incision of the plastron. 2. Vesicovaginal dissection. 3. Vesicouterine dissection. 4. Opening the paravesical space. 5. Enlarging the space with a finger. 6. Dissection of the tendinous arch, followed by placing the suspending threads. 7. Dissection, followed by placing the retrosymphyseal suspending threads. 8. Suspension of the plastron.

Guide to the reader

1. Recognise the indications and counter-indications for the plastron technique.
2. Describe all the operative actions involved in mobilisation of the bladder.
3. Describe the technique for opening of the paravesical fossae and dissection of the tendinous arches.
4. Detail the chronology of the actions related to the plastron, to vaginal hysterectomy and to Campbell's procedure in case of associated treatments.
5. Know how to use an alternative for the case of a defective tendinous arch.
6. Find the anatomic location of the ureter during the main operative stages and be aware of the risks encountered.

Cystocele treatment via the vaginal approach by the plastron technique, as developed by Gilles Crépin, is designed for the vaginal treatment of prolapse with a major cystocoele in menopausal women.
The condition for realisation of the plastron technique is the existence of excess tissue from the anterior vaginal wall, allowing the fashioning of a vaginal flap. Remaining attached to the bladder, this flap will be suspended then enclosed during anterior colporrhaphy upon vaginal closure. This highlights both the advantages and inconveniences of the technique. Since the tissue used is of autologous origin, it will not be rejected. However, the plastron can not be realised in pre-menopausal women, due to the risk of a secondary mucocele. Even in patients under substitutional hormonal treatment, it is advisable to interrupt the treatment for 3 to 6 months in order to reduce the risks. The size of the plastron will depend on the amount of excess vaginal tissue present and, in case of a moderate cystocele, its size will be limited, even though this risks vaginal narrowing. This simple technique unites the advantages brought about by lateral cystocele treatment via lateral suspension to the pelvic fascias' tendinous arches, and by central median cystocele treatment by a reinforcement resulting from the multiplication of the subvesical tissue layers.

The plastron technique is limited to:
– patients who are disturbed by their prolapse;
– patients who are fully informed about potential risks associated with the procedure;
– cystoceles that extend at least to the vulva;
– post-menopausal patients.

RELATED TECHNIQUES OR OPERATIVE ACTIONS

The surgical intervention resembles:
– vaginal culdoplasty techniques to enclose the vagina;
– paravaginal suspensions for suspension to the tendinous arches of the pelvic fascias;
– treatment of moderate cystocele according to Raz or Zimmern, using the four corners technique without enclosure of the vagina, but with suspension of the vaginal tissue to the abdominal aponeurosis.

Description

A typical procedure consists of a complete vaginal treatment of a prolapse, associating for the anterior stages a treatment of cystocele by plastron and Campbell's procedure in connection with a vaginal hysterectomy.

Positioning the Kocher forceps

The Kocher forceps are positioned on the plastron's four corners in relation to the anterior vaginal wall (*figure 16.2*). In order to determine their exact placement, one must, of course, verify the presence and extent of the excess of vaginal tissue. The plastron should be about 5 to 6 cm wide and 6 to 8 cm long. Its size cannot be reduced below 4 cm width and 5 cm height without also reducing its effectiveness. In case of a limited cystocele, following the forceps' positioning, one will have

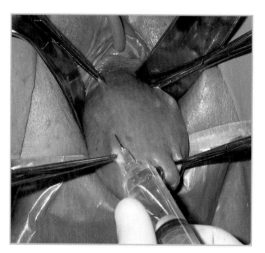

16.2 Kocher forceps in place, infiltration.

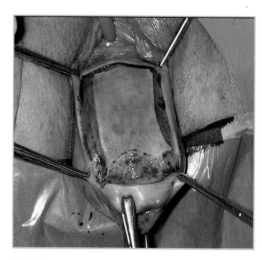

16.3 Plastron incision.

to examine the possibility of later performing vaginal closure in the absence of tension by bringing together the right and left Kocher forceps.

Infiltration

It is not necessary to infiltrate the plastron, which will remain attached to the bladder without being dissected. However, 50 to 60 cm3 of a mixture of adrenalin-containing Xylocaïne and physiologic serum will be infiltrated into the laterovesical space, as far as inside the vaginal pouches and paravesical fossae.

Incision of the plastron

Having spread the Kocher forceps and put the uterine cervix under tension by the Museux' forceps whenever possible, a firm incision is carried out between the Kocher forceps. Two Allis' forceps are then placed on the plastron's right and left side, grasping the whole of the incised vaginal section. The incision is completed at the forceps' position. By lifting and separating the Allis' forceps, the dissection space between the vaginal tissue and the bladder will be opened (*figure 16.3*).

Vesicovaginal dissection

Using a cold scalpel, the dissection will be commenced either on the right or left (*figure 16.4*), by lifting the homolateral Allis' forceps and opening the space between the bladder (held with a toothed forceps) and the vagina (stretched by the Allis' forceps). This dissection can be performed using a cold scalpel, since the bladder is displaced by the infiltration (*figure 16.5*).

Dissection to the vaginal pouches

The dissection is laterally extended as far as the vaginal pouches at the level of the bladder. In fact, the dissection space must be sufficiently large to provide a correct view and allow opening of the paravesical spaces. If one wishes to reposition

During the bladder's lateral dissection there is risk of damage the ureter, especially in case of a large cystocele where the ureter will also be externalised. However, this dissection is indispensable for moving the bladder upwards without leaving the bladder's lateral sides attached and thus risking postoperative bending of the ureter. In case of a large cystocele, it is, therefore, advisable to palpate the ureter between two finger before continuing with the lateral dissection.

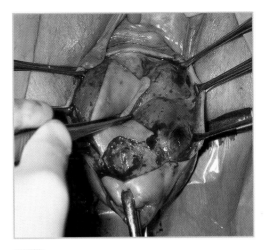

16.4 Left lateral vesical dissection.

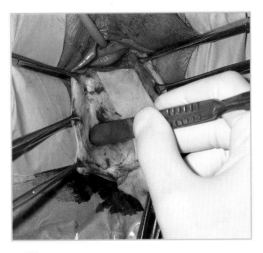

16.5 Right vesical dissection with the scalpel's handle.

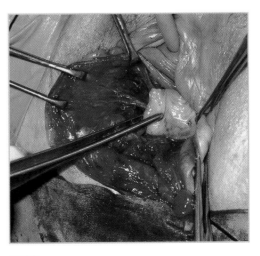

16.6 Visualisation of the dissection space by placing the bladder under tension.

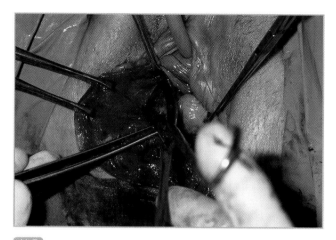

16.7 Section of the lateral adherences, opening of the paravesical space.

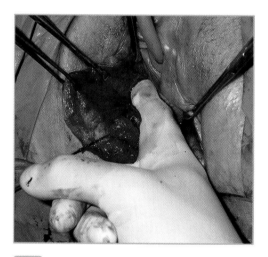

16.8 Dissection extended with a finger: opening the paravesical space.

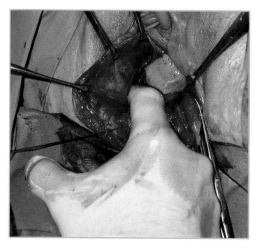

16.9 Enlarging the paravesical space with the help of a finger.

the bladder during its suspension, it is even more important to completely mobilise it without leaving any vaginal attachments that would pull it towards the sacrospinous ligaments via the Richter suspension. Initiated with a cold scalpel, the dissection is pursued with scissors or, the easier variant, with a finger covered with a compress (*figure 16.7*).

Execution of the vaginal colpohysterectomy

In case of an associated hysterectomy, the paravesical fossae will not be immediately opened. This eliminates risk of bleeding into the operative field originating from the dissection spaces. The complete vaginal hysterectomy procedure will now be carried out as described. A complete dissection is however carried out between the vesical base and uterine cervix and uterine isthmus on the median line, and with the suspending ligaments laterally.

For the case of post-hysterectomy prolapse
In the absence of hysterectomy, perfect mobility of the bladder with respect to the vaginal fundus is achieved by performing extensive dissection between the bladder and vaginal scar.

Repositioning the Allis' forceps

The hysterectomy having been accomplished, three Allis' forceps are repositioned on both sides along the anterior vaginal incision. The bladder's lateral dissection plane is thus revealed at the level of the vaginal pouches. The Allis' forceps are lifted on one side and the dissection extended laterally until the paravesical fossae are open.

Opening the paravesical fossae

After having liberated the bladder laterally, the paravesical fossae are opened with dissection forceps that are held in contact with the pubic symphysis, behind the vaginal pouch (*figure 16.7*). The closed scissors are oriented towards the Retzius space at the 2 o'clock position to the left and the 10 o'clock position to the right, the pelvic aponeurosis is perforated and the space is then opened by spreading the scissors' blades. One can now introduce a finger into this space in order to make sure that this space's opening has been effective (*figure 16.8*). This is confirmed if the finger can easily reach the top of the Retzius' space. The index finger is now used to enlarge the opening, laterally brushing the pubic branch (*figure 16.9*). The opening is extended laterally, away from the median line, until a narrow retractor can be placed inside the paravesical fossa.

Dissection of the pelvic fascias' tendinous arches

This retractor is positioned such that it pushes the bladder towards the median line, thus facilitating access to the pelvic wall (figure 16.10). As the assistant surgeon spreads the Allis' forceps, one can palpate the pelvic fascia's tendinous arches with the index finger. In order to perform the correct gesture for its palpation, it is indispensable to visualise its position with a sketched drawing. This tendinous arch is defined by a densification of the pelvic aponeurosis linking the dorsal part of the obturator's orifice and the ischial spine. Difficulties are sometimes encountered due to the previous collapse of the pelvic aponeurosis that is required during radical opening of the paravesical fossa. This collapse can result in "detaching" the tendinous arches from the pelvic wall, which makes their palpation an extremely delicate procedure.

To simplify the search and limit the dissection that would be required for locating the ischial spine, one can begin by identifying the inner edge of the obturator's orifice before searching its dorsal elongation via the tendinous arch. In fact, the fleshiest and most stable part of the tendinous arch lies in proximity to the obturator's orifice where the tendinous arches of the pelvic fascia and of the levator muscles mix. The finger must pass outside the tendinous arch, leaving it in contact with the pelvic wall. Sometimes, however, individualisation of the tendinous arch is impossible, or its structure too fine to be useful for suspension. Rather than accepting a suspension of insufficient stability, it is advisable to apply one of the alternatives briefly discussed at the end of this chapter.

Having palpated the tendinous arches on the pelvic wall, one now places the suspension threads.

Positioning the suspension threads

The plastron is a vaginal flap, which must be suspended in a harmonious manner in order to be efficient. Three suspension points are put into place both on the right and on the left. The first suspension point that will suspend the plastron's upper corner is put into place beneath the pubic branch and makes use of the thread used for suspension of the uterosacral ligament during Campbell's procedure. The other two points, suspending the median part and lower corner, respectively, are placed within the fleshy pre-spinal part of the pelvic fascia's tendinous arch (figure 16.11).

The passage of the first stitch on the patient's left side is technically easier. Having moved the vaginal pouch out of the way with the help of the Allis' forceps, the needle is presented by the needle-holder, perpendicular to the lower part of the pubic rami (figure 14.1). The needle is grazes along the osseous branch for 1 to 2 cm before being grasped with an empty needle-holder.

Bladder injury
In the case of a bladder injury one must:
– confirm the diagnosis with an intravesical blue-dye test;
– suture in one plane after identification of the openings in the bladder;
– verify the suture's tightness by another blue colour test;
– place a urinary catheter with free drainage for at least 5 days, in consideration of the proximal dissections' importance; duration is related to the wound's position and size.
In the case of a large wound it could be necessary to check the healing by cystography before removal of the catheter on day 8.

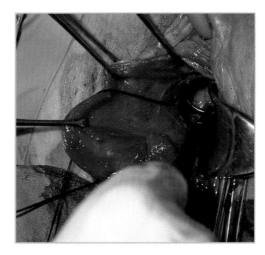

16.10 Retractor holding back the bladder, positioning of the suspension threads.

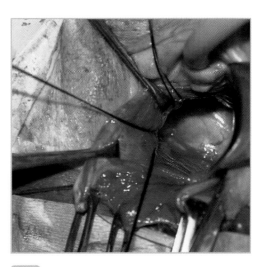

16.11 Positioning the suspension threads on the pelvic fascias' tendinous arches.

One must make sure that the needle is not transfixing at the vaginal level. If one encounters difficulties in placing this stitch, one can place the Allis' forceps at the level of the vaginal pouch in order to facilitate its location. A right-handed surgeon will pass the needle from front to back for the left stitch, and from back to front for the right stitch, the risk of transfixion being more elevated on the right side. Once the stitch has been placed, its stability must be tested by applying firm traction.

Placing the second and third threads requires more dexterity as the available space will be more restricted. The index finger will again be used to localise the pelvic fascia's tendinous arch and guide the needle's entry, rotation and exit. The procedure, therefore, relies on palpation and not on vision. Some surgeons use a type DFS or Endostitch stapler for this procedure. Although it facilitates placement of the suspension points, the apparatus' considerable cost has limited its distribution. Furthermore, experience allows rapid and easy positioning of the threads in most cases. The difficulty lies in correctly placing the needle and grasping it at its exit point with a needle-holder under the mere guidance of the index finger. The retractor, possibly supported by the addition of a gauze swab, protects the bladder, and the thread must exclusively take hold at the tendinous arch. Of course, one must test the stability of this hold before placing the next thread.

At this point of the procedures, the threads are not passed through the plastron so as not to close the dissection space and risk tangling the threads. We, therefore, advise to keep the threads long and successively organise them on the Allis' forceps (figure 16.12). The subsymphyseal thread is passed onto the upper forceps, and so forth.

Haemorrhage

In the case of a haemorrhage originating in the dissection space of the paravesical fossae one must:
– reposition the retractors, search for localised bleeding, especially in the laterovesical direction;
– locally compress for several minutes using several compresses;
If diffuse bleeding persists after having put the suspensions under tension and having performed local compression, one will place a urinary probe for 24 hours (the bladder will be filled with 200 cm^3 and clamped for 2 hours postoperatively), as well as an intravaginal gauze drain, also for 24 hours.

Plastron suspension

Once the six suspension threads are in place, gauze drain and retractor are removed. Haemostasis, usually consisting of a diffuse bleeding originating from the paravesical fossae, is verified. We advise a counting of the compresses at this point, so that the suspension will not have to be dismounted at the end of the intervention in order to retrieve a compress forgotten in a paravesical fossa (as happened to us once). In case of

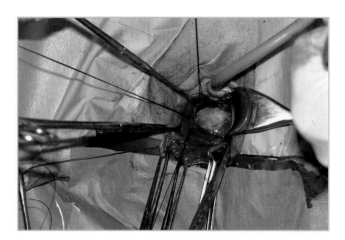

16.12 Three threads put into place on the right.

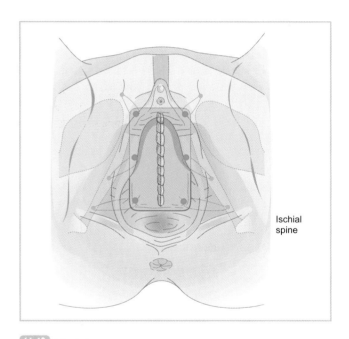

Ischial spine

16.13 Final view.

localised bleeding, a haemostasis stitch is put into place. One can now pass the threads through the plastron. The threads are placed, but, in order to facilitate placement of the subsequent threads, are not yet put under tension. The vaginal passage of the thread can and must be of substantial depth, taking hold of the total vaginal thickness with an "X" stitch over a minimum of 1 cm. Once the six suspension threads have been passed through the plastron, they are progressively put under tension. One must avoid bringing the plastron into direct contact with the tendinous arches as well as overtightening the threads. Furthermore, it is advisable to successively tighten the right and left points at each level in order to obtain symmetric tension.

Anterior vaginal closure

Once the plastron has been suspended, the compresses are counted before beginnning the vaginal closure. If the uterosacral ligaments are crossed subsymphyseally as during Campbell's technique, the two uterosacral ligaments will have to be suspended before cutting the suspension threads. The suspension threads are cut short and saggital closure of the vagina is achieved with a crossed overcasting suture as far as the vaginal floor (*figure 16.13*).

ALTERNATIVES

Alternative in the case of deficient tendinous arches

In our experience, in about 5% of the cases the tendinous arches are too thin to permit a solid suspension of the plastron. Two elegant solutions can be applied to circumvent this problem:
– suspension to the abdominal aponeurosis;
– suspension across the obturator orifice.

Suspension to the abdominal aponeurosis

The first of these solutions consists in transfering the threads across Retzius' space in order to suspend them on the abdominal aponeurosis. Due to the dissection of the paravesical fossae, the Retzius' space can easily be dissected with a finger. A Stamey needle can be passed from top to bottom to successively bring the four suspension threads upwards. These will be knotted two-by-two above the abdominal aponeurosis inside a short incision measuring 5 mm. The tension applied will be moderate, so as to avoid over-correcting, this technique's principal risk.

Suspension across the obturator's orifice

The second solution consists of suspensing the threads to the median pelvic aponeurosis at the level of the obturator orifice. As in the above-described method, a short incision measuring 5 mm is realised. With the help of the Stamley needle, the two threads are successively retrieved on either side and knotted inside the incision. The needle's path across the obturator's orifice will be described in detail in the chapter discussing the treatments for urinary incontinence (*cf.* chapter 25).

Alternative in the case of less extensive cystocele or for premenopausal women

We have discussed the limitations of the indications for cystocele treatment by the plastron technique. A moderate cystocele must be treated during vaginal-approach procedures treatment via the vaginal approach, otherwise there is a high risk of relapse. In the same fashion, in premenopausal woman there is an elevated risk of a secondary mucocele if vaginal tissue is enclosed.

During planning of the procedure one has the choice between the following three solutions:
– absence of treatment of the cystocele: this decision increases the risk of relapse if one performs a posterior suspension and the cystocele is large. Thus, for treatment of prolapse of the vaginal floor according to Richter, secondary cystocele have been documented in more than 15 % of the cases;
– prolapse cure via an abdominal approach with anterior and posterior prostheses, as well as ligamentopexy; without a doubt, this is the best validated and most prudent approach to follow in such a situation. It guarantees good long term results and that can, in most cases, be achieved by laparoscopy;
– the use of heterologous or synthetic material; for vaginal surgeons, this represents a great temptation... One might produce a plastron from autologous or heterologous tissue, such as the fascia lata, or a prosthesis of animal origin. A synthetic prosthesis, such as Prolene, can also be used (*cf.* chapter 23). However, these materials are just now being validated for their application to vaginal surgery, and we can not advise their use except within the context of clinical studies.

TYPICAL AFTER-EFFECTS OF THE OPERATION

The plastron rarely causes persisting pain.

Transitory postoperative urinary retention is frequent: do not forget to verify the mictional residue, even in the absence of an associated treatment of urinary incontinence. Repeated catheterisation is sometimes required over several days.

In 10 % of the cases, the routine check-up will reveal a postoperative granuloma – which can cause leucorrhoea and vesical instability – resulting from an apparent suspension thread. The treatment is based on disinfection by insertion of a pessory and the result is evaluated two months later. If the problem persists, the thread will be resected during a consultation.

CHAPTER 17

Posterior operational stages – Suspension of the vaginal vault according to Richter

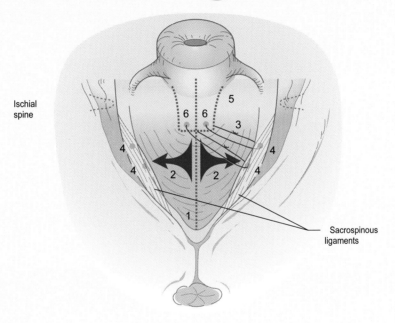

Ischial
spine

Sacrospinous
ligaments

17.1 *Summary sketch.*
1. Posterior longitudinal incision. 2. Rectovaginal incision and opening of the paravesical fossae.
3. Dissection of the sacrospinous ligaments, especially on the left. 4. Two non-resorbable threads
passed through the ligament. 5. Creation of two vaginal strips. 6. Threading the strips with suspension
threads.

Guide to the reader

1. Identify the different operational stages for dissection of the sacrospinous ligament.
2. Indicate the traps and complications this dissection might entail.
3. Describe the act allowing the needle's passage through the ligament.
4. Describe the technique of vaginal suspension and the order of events, commencing with vaginal closure.

*T*he technique and indications for this
intervention, originally described as a vaginal
approach for the treatment of post-hysterectomy
prolapses, have undergone many adaptations. The
principle, however, has remained unchanged, and
is based on suspension of the vaginal vault to the
right or left sacrospinous ligament via a suture
thread passed through the vaginal wall on one
end and the ligament's width at the other end.
By suspending the vaginal floor to a strong
ligament, this vaginal operation can be compared
to the principle behind prevertebral ligamentopexy
performed via an abdominal approach.
This procedure has now become the key
technique of all prolapse treatments via a vaginal
approach, and is usually associated with anterior
and posterior operational procedures.

TECHNICAL VARIATIONS

In contrast to the chromed catgut used in this technique's
early description, the thread applied today is usually non-
resorbable.

Some surgeons advise to always perform this procedure
bilaterally.

Similarly, some surgeons prefer to realise the passage through
the ligament in a blind fashion, orienting themselves by palpation and us of specific materials (staples, Endostitch...).

DESCRIPTION

We will describe the suspension technique according to
Richter, including some alterations that we have integrated in
the procedure. The technique is either applied for prolapses of
the vaginal floor without an association with anterior stages in
the absence of a cystocele, or for complete prolapse treatment
following closure of the anterior vaginal wall.

In keeping with Richter's initial description, we perform a
unilateral suspension to the sacrospinous ligaments. Due to
our operation theatre's organisation and video retransmission
we perform this suspension on the patient's left ligament – of
course, this does not represent a recommendation.

Vaginal infiltration

The intervention begins with the placement of three Kocher
forceps in stages along the median part of the posterior vaginal
wall, the highest being placed above the vaginal vault, or, if the
uterine cervix is to be conserved one cm beneath the cervix;
the lowest of the forceps is positioned at the level of the cutaneomucous division, about 2 cm from the vulvar orifice; the
third forceps is positioned halfway between the other two. By
applying tension to theses forceps, one can completly expose
the complete incision line. The intramuscular infiltration consists of about 30 ml of 1% adrenalin-containing Xylocaïne and
30 ml physiological serum. The injection is performed under
the vaginal thickness, at the level of the line of incision, and
laterally to the rectum, as far as the pararectal spaces.

Attention: the infiltration prepares for the entirety of the
following dissection. It is, therefore, mandatory that it be
performed precisely in the dissection plane. One must:
– be careful not to perform the infiltration too superficially
under the mucous membrane;
– avoid performing the infiltration too deeply, e.g. inside the
rectal wall, especially during lateral pararectal infiltration.

Median vaginal incision

The vaginal incision is achieved with a cold scalpel by
sectioning the vaginal wall. Two separate incisions are
performed between the Kocher forceps (*figure 17.2*).

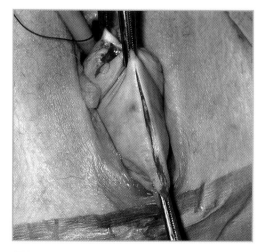

17.2 Posterior vaginal incision, Kocher forceps
in place.

Positioning the Allis' forceps

The eight Allis' forceps can now be positioned. They take hold of the entire vaginal wall on either side, and divergent traction, applied by the assistant surgeons, exposes the dissection plane. The Kocher forceps are removed before commencing the incision below the middle Kocher forceps (figure 17.3).

Rectovaginal dissection

While the Allis' forceps are being pulled away from each other, one performs the recto-vaginal dissection by incising the infiltrated plane between vagina and rectum with a cold scalpel (*figures 17.4 and 17.5*). This incision is extended by counter-later-ally spreading the rectum with a toothless forceps. The dissection can easily be extended with a finger (*figures 17.6 and 17,7*), and opening of the pararectal trenches starts at the upper end, at the 4 o'clock position on the patient's left side and on the 8 o'clock position on her right side. This opening is achieved without

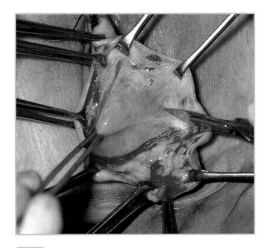

17.5 Left rectovaginal dissection.

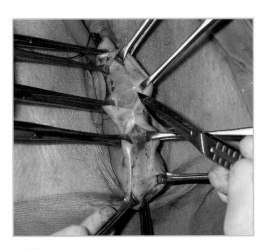

17.3 Incision completed after positioning the Allis' forceps.

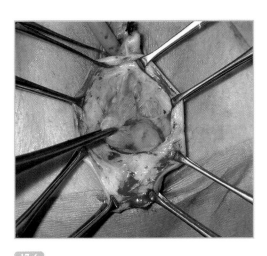

17.6 Rectovaginal dissection completed.

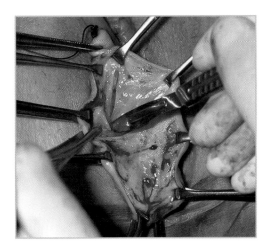

17.4 Right rectovaginal dissection.

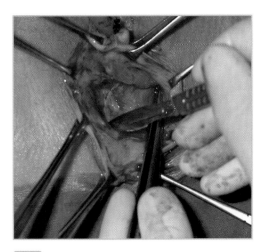

17.7 Liberating the lower part of the rectum.

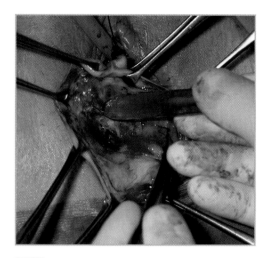

17.8 Dissection with the scalpel's lateral handle.

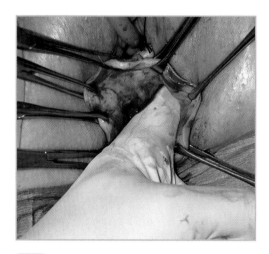

17.9 Beginning the opening of the left pararectal fossa.

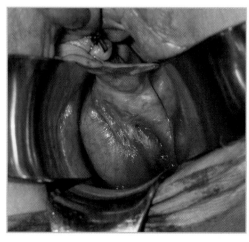

17.10 Positioning the three retractors: dissection space, rectum, levator muscle.

exerting any force. It is enlarged by rubbing the rectum's lateral part as far as the levator muscles with a finger (*figures 17.8 and 17.9*). For the incision's lower part, it is often necessary to lift the rectum with a toothed forceps in order to liberate its lateral and lower attachments. This additional dissection has to be performed before placing the retractors permitting the dissection of the sacrospious ligament, so that pushing back the rectum with the large retractor does not result in a rectal wound from dilacerations at the level of its lateral attachments.

However, the procedure should not be continued in a blind fashion by finger dissection as far as the ligament; we prefer to place some retractors so as to be able to continue the dissection under visual control.

Positioning the retractors

First, the posterior retractor is put into place so that the posterior Allis' forceps can be removed. One then brings the small lateral retractor in contact with the levator muscle. The left Allis' retractors can now be removed before placing the large Breitski retractor and removing the remaining Allis' forceps. This improves the retractors' mobility, thus allowing enlargement of the operative field (*figure 17.10*).

One must ascertain that the left retractor does not reach beyond the levator muscle, masking the dissection space.
One must also make sure that the right retractor correctly holds back the rectum. If necessary, a gauze drain can be placed so that the rectum can be pushed away more efficiently.

Opening the pararectal space

It is necessary to visualise the limit between the levator muscle and rectum (*figure 17.11*). This limit is easily identifiable if it

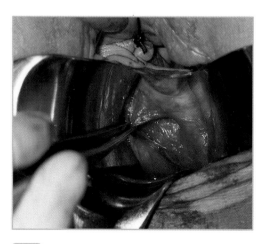

17.11 Continuing the opening of the left pararectal fossa.

is correctly displayed by the assistant surgeons' retractors. It is recognisable by prerectal fatty tissue belonging to an adherent portion of the levator muscle. This space can easily be opened using a little "nut" held with a Jean-Louis Faure forceps, which, when rubbed against the muscle from front to back, pushes back the rectum (*figure 17.12*). Once the dissection has significantly progressed, the retractors are repositioned and the dissection continued. In order to open the dissection space further, one can apply divergent traction on two forceps. The gauze drain is positioned more deeply on the rectum before repositioning the retractors. The dissection is performed in contact with the levator muscle (*figure 17.13*): this is a useful point of orientation that will always lead to the sacrospinous ligament. This dissection is carried out away from the ischial spine, which should never be within the dissection space, even though it can sometimes be detected by palpation.

Attention: in the case of prior myorraphy of the levator muscles, this dissection plane can be difficult and one must be careful:
– to pass through the remainder of the levator muscles by dissecting a plane ending below the ligament;
– not to insure the rectum wound during the course of the dissection.

Dissection of the sacrospinous ligament

The ligament itself is deeply positioned, and, if there is any doubt the extent of the remaining dissection, it might be useful to evaluate this by removing the retractors. It becomes visible as a whitish membrane (*figure 17.14*) covering the posterior fibres of the levator muscle before spreading out across the pelvic wall (*figure 17.15*). A reinforcing of this pelvic aponeurosis can be seen at the lower part of the levator muscle.

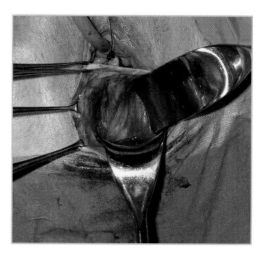
17.13 View of the left levator muscle's dissection.

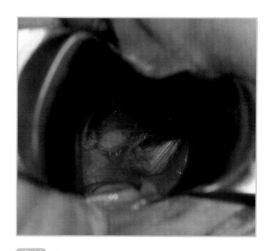
17.14 Sacro-epinal ligament under some adherences.

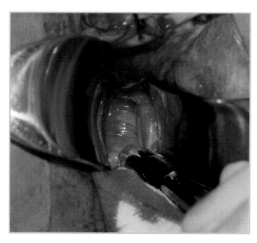
17.12 Dissection of the levator muscle with a small "nut".

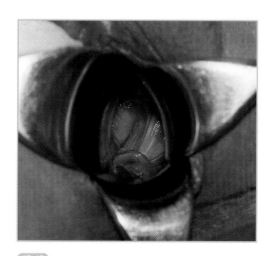
17.15 Left sacro-epinal ligament.

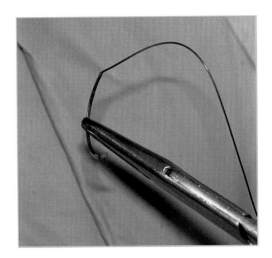

17.16 Grasping the suspension needle.

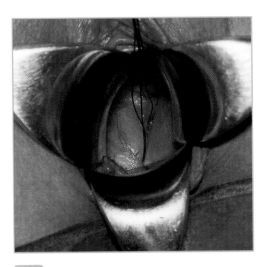

17.17 Having placed the thread, the left levator muscle's haemostasis is verified.

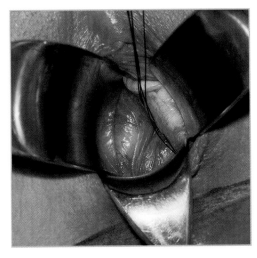

17.18 Verifying the rectum's haemostasis.

Attention: should the ligament not present this characteristic aspect there will be a risk of:
– dissecting beyond the sacrospinous ligament;
– major haemorrhage.
In case of doubt, remove the lateral retractor and palpate the ligament, which, even if not always visible, should always be palpable. If the ligament is not palpable, palpate the counterlateral ligament and choose the most favourable side.

Passing the needle through the ligament

The passing of the needle through the ligament is, without a doubt, the operation's most delicate moment. The ligament's deep position; its inherent thinness and its position along the wall; the narrow dissection space limiting the radius of needle rotation, and the proximity to the rectum all represent limiting factors. It is further recommended to pass the needle from back to front in order to prevent injury from the needle point to the vascular pedicles that are close to the ischial spine, should the needle deviate from the intended path (figure 17.16).

One will now see why such a large number of forceps are being used, including some that are applied outside the context of their original intent, in order to facilitate this action. With a bit of exercise, it will always be possible, and above all easier and cheaper, to pass a thread through the ligament. We prefer to place two non-resorbable plaited threads in order to prevent rupture or accidental release of one of the sutures during the subsequent manipulation.

In order to facilitate the thread's placement, the needle will be mounted on a needle-holder, and held such that the tip points towards the left and towards the operator, so that it can be passed from back to front (figure 17.16). It is first passed behind the ligament and then pushed towards the surgeon. As soon as the tip becomes visible, it is gripped by a second needle-holder, without letting go of the first. Following the same procedure a second thread is put into place.

Controlling haemostasis and the hold's stability

Firm traction must be applied on the thread in order to verify the hold's stability. In case of doubt, do not hesitate to place a new suture. Once the stability has been confirmed, haemostasis is verified. To this end, one will first ensure the absence of haemorrhages along the levator muscle without moving the gauze pad (figure 17.17) before putting the lateral retractor back into place and ablating the gauze pad. By progressively removing the large retractor one can now examine the complete rectal wall and especially its vascularisation; sometimes lesions are found above the opening of the pararectal fossa (*figure 17.18*). Such vascular lesions are rare, however, and the three retractors can now be removed and Allis' forceps put back into place in order to continue the intervention.

One might be satisfied with the Richter suspension but, after having efficiently suspended the vaginal vault, we believe it is indispensable to complete the process with effective support of the vaginal wall's lower part by myorrhaphy of the levator muscles.

Haemorrhage

In the case of a operative haemorrhage originating in the pararectal fossa, pressure is applied with a compress to the wound and the retractors are replaced in order to obtain a good viewing.

If a localised haemorrhage persists after compression, a haemostasis stitch will be carried out.

In the case of a strong haemorrhage of the pudendal pedicle that is not accessible for haemostasis, the compression is prolonged.

If necessary, arterial embolisation will be performed with radiology. In the absence of embolisation, a gauze drain is put into place (cf. Mickulicz) for haemostasis by compression. A follow-up procedure is planned 48 hours later for removal of the gauze drain and verification of haemostasis.

Myorrhaphy of the levator muscles

This will be described in more detail in the following chapter, but it is important to mention that the vaginal vault is never suspended according to Richter's technique in the absence of an associated myorrhaphy of the levator muscles.

Verifying rectal integrity

Myorrhaphy of the levator muscles is accompanied by a systematic verification of rectal integrity by rectal examination. The main goal is to verify that threads have not transfixed the

Rectal injury
These are of several types:
– Injury caused during recto-vaginal dissection, or a serous injuries on the proximal lateral or ventral segment;
– Injury caused by the positioning of the retractors: at the lower part of the dissection of the pararectal space.
In the case of doubt, perform a rectal examination, as well as a blue dye test.
In the case of a rectal injury, it will be closed with a simple overcast suture and the quality of the seal verified by applying another blue colour test. The patient is put onto a residue-free list

rectum. This rectal examination does not replace verification of the rectum's integrity as required during the check for haemostasis (see above).

The start of vaginal closure and determining the point of suspension

Before beginning vaginal closure one must determine the position of the new vaginal fundus. Its exact location is determined by the point of symmetry between the anterior and posterior walls; hysterectomy, resection of the anterior vaginal floor and an efficient suspension, even in the absence of a resection, will always alter the position of the vaginal vault.

Identifying its position is important—once the position of the vaginal-vault suspension is determined, one can perform a preliminary closing of the vaginal floor up to the selected position. To do this, the vaginal incision's edges are grasped with two Allis' forceps at a position that appears adequate (*figure 17.19*), and the operation's end result is simulated by bringing the two forceps in contact with the ligament, which, of course, pulls the remaining forceps upwards, too. The anatomical correction will be complete and perfectly symmetrical if the suspension point is well selected. Should the correction be asymmetrical, the forceps are repositioned until a positioning is found that permits a symmetrical anatomical correction.

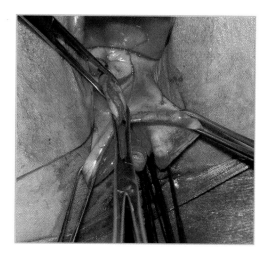

17.19 Identification of the vaginal floor before vaginal closure.

Suspension of the vaginal vault: the technique of the vaginal strips

We have seen that, by this stage of the operation, the threads are in place at the level of the sacrospinous ligament.

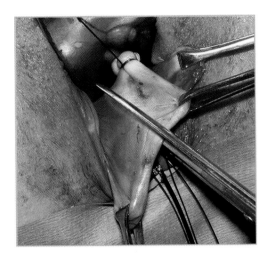

17.20 Right vaginal strip.

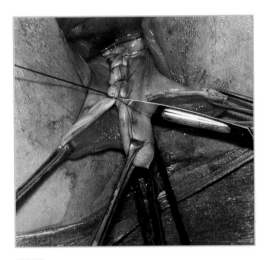

17.21 Removal of the left strip's epidermis.

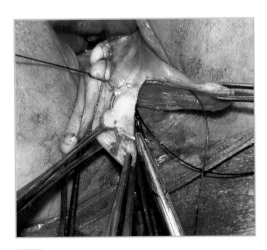

17.22 Left vaginal strip held with the needle.

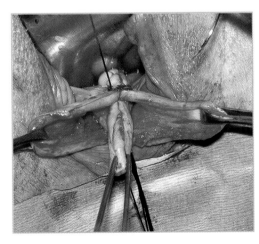

17.23 Vaginal closure, and enclosing of the two vaginal strips.

Vaginal suspension is more delicate, since it must be just as firm but can only be performed on the vaginal tissue itself, and it cannot transfix this tissue if non-resorbing thread is used. This suspension, therefore, represents the weak point of the overall suspension. This is why, inspired by the Bologna intervention for the cure of urinary incontinence (*cf.* chapter 28), we perform this suspension using two strips fashioned of vaginal tissue. This technique was described by Gilles Crépin and consists of the preparation of two vaginal strips, after deciding on the positioning of the vaginal floor. A surface of about 2 cm by 3 cm of the vaginal floor will provide a base of implantation for the strips (*figure 17.20*).

Before realising the suspension, one begins vaginal closure as far as the representative position of the future vaginal floor. The thread is simply kept stretched, and about 2 cm further up, the vaginal section is grasped on either side by an Allis' forceps that is pulled towards the midline. Using scissors, one merely now has to merely section a 2-by-3-cm-long strip with a wide implantation base relative to the reference point for the vaginal floor (*figure 17.20*). The epidermis is ablated by superficially scratching the strip (*figure 17.21*) before piercing it with a needle carrying one of the threads passed through the sacrospinous ligament (*figure 17.22*). The same action is performed contralaterally.

Vaginal closure and putting the suspensions under tension

Before putting the Richter suspension threads under tension, it is recommended to carry out a nearly complete closure of the vaginal incision, because the vaginal ascension due to the suspension will render this act extremely delicate. The continuous suture applied for the closure grasps the incision's edges and progressively encloses the suspension strips (*figure 17.23*). Once the crossed overcast suture leaves just enough space for a finger to pass, the threads are put under tension (*figures 17.24* and *17.25*). Tension will be applied to one thread after the other,

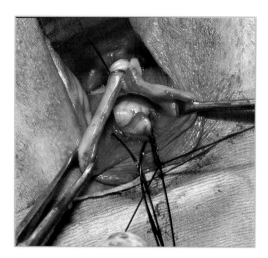

17.24 Continuation of vaginal closure, vaginal strips enclosed.

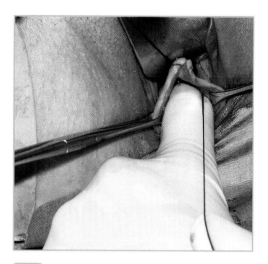

17.25 Putting the threads under tension, 2 cm from the vulva.

while the finger follows the knot inside the pararectal fossauntil it reaches the sacrospinous ligament but without tension, bringing the vaginal strip almost in contact with the ligament. The same procedure is followed for the second thread. In case of an associated myorrhaphy, the myorrhaphy thread is also knotted before finishing the overcast suture of the vaginal closure. At this stage, the suspension threads can be cut short.

Once vaginal closure has been achieved, haemostasis is again verified, especially as far as good concurrence of the edges of the vaginal incision is concerned. The compresses will be counted once again before carrying any required action for urinary matters.

The threads have been passed about 2 cm from the ischial spine (figure 17.26). The result is illustrated in figure 17.27.

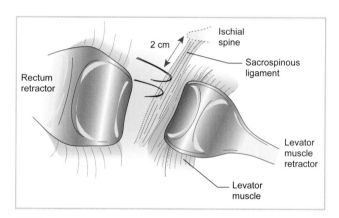

17.26 Position of the suspension thread.

TYPICAL POSTOPERATIVE CONSIDERATIONS

Characteristic consequences of the operation require:
– An average of 3 days hospitalisation;
– perineal pains over several weeks: analgesic treatment, support pillow for the sitting position;
– increased pains while sitting, during effort and bowel movement;
– treatment to prevent postoperative constipation.

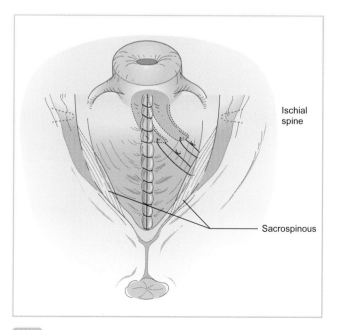

17.27 The surgical procedures' final result.

CHAPTER 18

Posterior operational stages – Myorrhaphy of the levator muscles

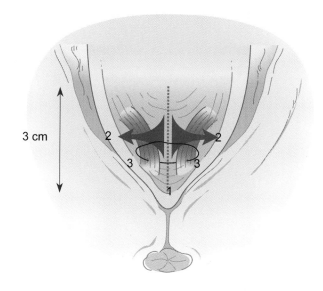

18.1 *Summary sketch.*
1. Posterior vaginal incision. 2. Rectovaginal dissection and beginning of the paravesical fossae.
3. Approach of the levator muscle above the vulvar bifurcation.

Guide to the reader

1. Indicate the order of stages for myorrhaphy of the levator muscles.
2. Name the different techniques applied when performing the procedure in isolation or in association with a suspension according to Richter.
3. Determine the principal intraoperative risks, their prevention and treatment.

Myorrhaphy of the levator muscles is often considered as accessory to the treatment of prolapse because it is terminal. It nevertheless remains a fundamental technique for prolapse treatment via the vaginal approach. Its principle is based on the unification of the levator muscles' along the median line. This action favours improved supporting of the vagina in its lower region and reconstitution of the perineal central fibrous core, which is often impaired. This technique by itself is not sufficient for the treatment of a high rectocele, which will have to be treated by the association with a suspension of the vaginal vault according to Richter.

TECHNICAL VARIATIONS

The principal variations are based on:
– the association of a perineorrhaphy;
– the importance of the thickness of the hold on the muscles;
– the height of the point of unification of the muscles.
The technically easy character of this procedure is counter-balanced by the postoperative perineal pains that sometimes last for several weeks. This explains why one is often tempted to avoid performing this procedure wherever possible, or to at least reduce its morbidity by merely bringing together the pre-rectal fascias. However, scientific studies have not yet identified any reliable alternative. In our eyes it appears indispensable, especially in the case of suspension of the vaginal floor according to Richter either via a vaginal or an abdominal approach, to create a support by myorrhaphy of the levator muscles.

Although it usually provides an esthetical result, we never associate a perineorrhaphy, since we find that it is not physiological and even a cause for postoperative dyspareunia. Furthermore, the esthetical result of any correction of vulvar malformations, obtained in a patient positioned in a forced gynaecological position, seems doubtful, since the corrections are performed in a position that is far from natural. What is more, it is not based on any scientific data, while the morbidity resulting from this procedure has been well described.

DESCRIPTION

The procedure described here is an isolated myorrhaphy of the levator muscles.

Comment: this is usually performed during the posterior stages of a prolapse treatment via a vaginal approach, in association with suspension of the vaginal vault according to Richter. As indicated in chapter 17, myorraphy is performed after placing the threads on the sacrospinous ligaments and before commencing vaginal closure. The main technical difference between performing the procedure in isolation or in association with suspension of the vaginal vault according to Richter lies in the vaginal opening and in the extent of the rectovaginal dissection and dissection of the pararectal fossae.

Placing the Kocher forceps and vaginal infiltration of the posterior vaginal wall

In the absence of an associated suspension, this infiltration, just like the incision, is limited to the lower half of the posterior vaginal wall. Only two Kocher forceps are, therefore, necessary, one positioned halfway from the vaginal floor and the other about 2 cm from the vulvar bifurcation.

Vaginal incision and placing the Allis' forceps

Only two Allis' forceps are required on either side of the vaginal incision, together grasping the whole of the vaginal section.

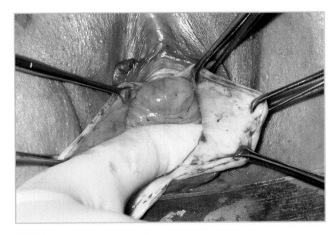

18.2 Rectovaginal dissection, incision's edges stretched with Allis' forceps.

Rectovaginal dissection and opening of the pararectal spaces

The dissection is performed as described in chapter 17 (Richter), but over a shorter distance (*figure 18.2*). The pararectal fossae are opened without trying to dissect as far as the sacrospinous ligament, which is most often not necessary. The dissection must be sufficient to allow rectal mobilisation and distancing of the rectum while placing the sutures inside the levator muscle.

Revealing the levator anal muscle

Due to the pathologies for which they are being treated, most patients on which myorrhaphy of the levator muscles is performed will present levator muscles that have suffered obstetric tearing. Their position is often modified and the muscle should not be sought along the median line, but more laterally, towards the back and the outside. The muscle becomes apparent by pulling on the Allis' forceps while the surgeon's finger holds back the rectum.

Passing the thread to the left

The slowly resorbable thread is introduced in the left side, the needle being inserted horizontally below the vaginal line of symmetry so as not to perforate the homolateral vaginal pouch. The needle is firmly pressed towards the lateral wall, so as to get hold of a maximum of muscle tissue before performing a U-turn and exiting at the back, in contact with the finger that pushes back the rectum (*figure 18.3*). The needle is retrieved with a second needle-holder. By pulling the Allis' forceps towards the midline, visually exposing the vaginal pouch, one verifies that the pouch was not taken up by the suture. One must also verify that the hold on the muscle is sufficient. To this end, traction is applied to the muscle in order to pull it towards the midline.

The needle is retrieved and one now begins with the patient's right side.

Passing the thread to the patient's right side

The needle is mounted on a needle-holder and presented perpendicular to the muscle at the farthest point possible, while holding the rectum back with the index finger of the left hand. The needle deeply penetrates the muscle towards the pelvic wall, before performing a rapid return, mirroring its passage on the left side, then being retrieved at the upper part of the levator muscle. Here, the needle exits right along the vagina (*figure 18.4*), and the risk of transfixing is much greater than on

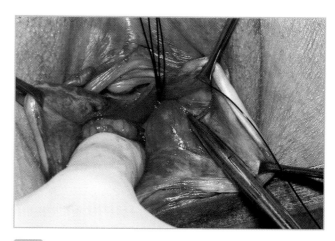

18.3   The needle is passed to the left, the index finger protecting and pushing back the bladder.

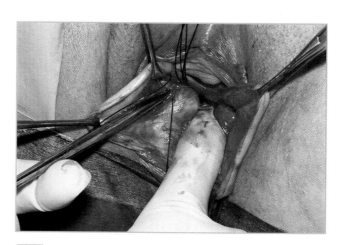

18.4   Passage to the right.

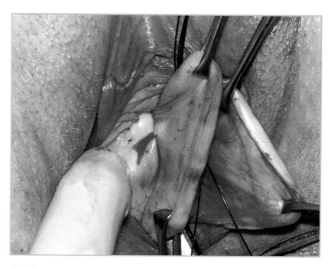

18.5   Transfixing suture inside the vaginal pouch.

the left. After having blocked the needle's exit with an empty needle-holder, the vaginal pouch's integrity is then examined before retrieving the needle. If the pouch has been transfixed (*figure 18.5*), the thread is repositioned. The procedure is repeated 1 to 2 cm above the vulvar orifice.

Verification of rectal integrity

At this point of the intervention, it is extremely easy to check for rectal integrity by rectal examination using a sterile finger cot. If the myorraphy suture is transfixing on one side, it will be removed and another one put into place, the passage of which will also have to be examined. It is not always easy to evaluate rectal integrity, given that the suture is in direct contact with the rectum and can easily be palpated, and combination of the glove and finger cot affects the sensations. It might, therefore, be helpful to glide the left hand's index finger between the thread and rectum in order to formally exclude an intrarectal passage.

Applying tension and vaginal closure

Where a suspension according to Richter is associated, one commences the vaginal closure before passing the suspension thread from the sacrospinous ligament to the level of the vaginal floor. In this case, the myorrhaphy is put under tension after the Richter's suspension, just before completing the vaginal closure.

If the myorrhaphy is performed in isolation, the stitches can directly be tightened without having to worry about an ill-timed vaginal ascent. The vaginal closure is then achieved with a single crossed overcast suture.

The operative stage is completed by controlling haemostasis and counting the compresses.

CHAPTER 19

Posterior operational stages – Douglassectomy

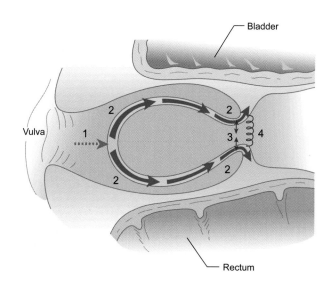

19.1 *Summary sketch.*
1. Incision of the elytrocele. 2. Dissection of the peritoneum. 3. Removal of the peritoneum. 4. Closing the elytrocele collar and rectovesical attachment.

Guide to the reader

1. Distinguish the different circumstances under which the procedure is performed in isolation, in association with a vaginal hysterectomy, or with a suspension of the vaginal vault according to Richter.
2. Identify the technique for dissection of the peritoneum.
3. Recognise the limits of elytrocele removal.

Douglassectomy represents an essential technique for treating an elytrocele. Since it is necessary, but not sufficient, it must be associated in a second operative stage with a suspension of the vaginal vault according to Richter. The procedure consists of a resection of the elytrocele's hernial sac via a vaginal approach. It is performed after a vaginal hysterectomy, in the case of a prolapse with the uterus in place, or represents the first stage in the case of a prolapse of the vaginal dome occurring as a consequence of hysterectomy.

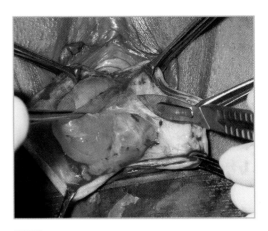

19.2 Rectovaginal dissection, liberating the elytrocele's sac.

VARIATIONS

The variations are risky:
– exclusion of the Douglas' pouch by layered purse-string sutures leading to the risk of peritoneal cysts;
– Richter suspension alone, leading to the risk of contralateral relapse if the Richter suspension was unilateral and the risk of persistant postural pains.

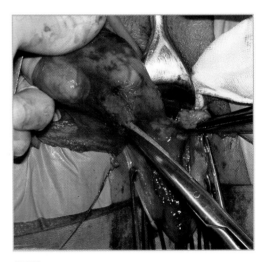

19.3 Peritoneal dissection with scissors (the sac is open).

DESCRIPTION

Douglassectomy begins by opening the Douglas' pouch. Since this was already achieved during hysterectomy, we will here describe a douglassectomy performed as a first stage of a treatment for post-hysterectomy vaginal prolapse.

The procedure is either preceded by an associated cystocele treatment, or one considers the elytrocele treatment and secondary suspension according to Richter sufficient. In the first scenario, cystocele treatment represents the first stage of the intervention and, since the elytrocele cure is only performed after anterior vaginal closure, the technique is identical.

Attention: in the case of a post-hysterectomy prolapse, it is often difficult to pre-operatively determine, by clinical examination, the relative degrees of cystocele or elytrocele. In some cases, even a prolapse that is isolated from the vaginal floor can, at least partially, contain the bladder that is rotated across the hysterectomy scar. An echographic examination – eventually an MRI if included in a research protocol – and, above all, an operative evaluation by placement of a Béniqué probe are necessary to locate the bladder more precisely. The infiltration is performed as at the beginning of a Richter intervention, after having placed the Kocher forceps as described according the same protocol.

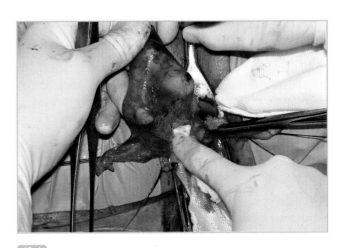

19.4 Peritoneal dissection with the help of a compress.

The incision and placement of the Allis' forceps allow the achievement of a complete opening of the posterior vaginal column.

The rectovaginal dissection commences in the same way, but, before opening the paravesical fossae, it is useful to dissect and resect the elytrocele's sac (*figure 19.2*). To this end, we will again perform a rectal examination in order to precisely locate the rectum if in doubt.

Having localised the rectum, the elytrocele's sac can be palpated between two fingers and subsequently opened to confirm the diagnosis.

Opening the elytrocele's sac will also allow the pushing back of any intestines before grasping the peritoneum with a heart-shaped forceps on its anterior and posterior parts.

Elytrocele dissection is completed.

By introducing a finger into the elytrocele pocket one can dissect the peritoneum as far up as possible, reaching the rectum dorsally and the bladder ventrally in the region where the peritoneum can no longer be detached (*figures 19.3 and 19.4*).

One must, at this stage, resect the peritoneal sac before considering peritoneal closure. This closure will be much facilitated if one takes the precaution to position four orientation marks in the peritoneal corners, above the resection limit, before resecting the peritoneum (*figure 19.5*). Without this precaution, there is a considerable risk to find oneself looking for the retracted peritoneal edges. To avoid this, four Kocher forceps are positioned on the peritoneum before resecting the excess peritoneum with thin scissors (*figure 19.5*).

The subvesical and prerectal peritoneum having been marked by the Kocher forceps, a purse-string suture is realised with a 2/0 resorbable thread. This closure permits a radical douglassectomy in association with a rectovesical approach, diminishing the risk of possible recurrence (*figures 19.6 and 19.7*).

The intervention can now be continued with a Richter suspension, as described in chapter 17.

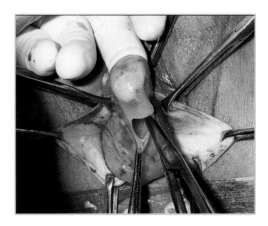

19.5 Peritoneal section after placement of the position-marking forceps.

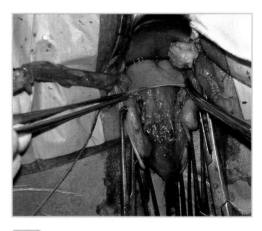

19.6 Remaining peritoneum after elytrocele resection.

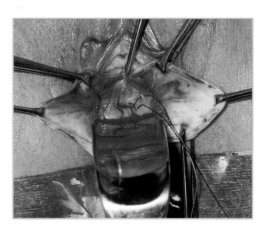

19.7 Peritoneal closure by rectovesical attachment.

CHAPTER 20

Posterior operational stages – Perineal repair according to Musset

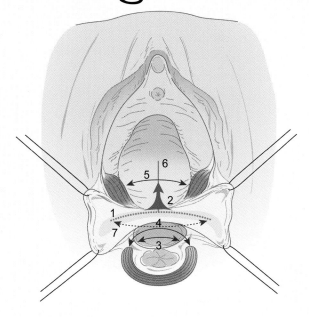

20.1 *Summary sketch.*
1. Incision. 2. Rectovaginal dissection. 3. Reconstruction of the anal canal. 4. Anal sphincteroplasty.
5. Low myorrhaphy of the levator muscles. 6. Posterior colporrhaphy. 7. Superficial perineorrhaphy.

Guide to the reader

1. Indicate the different operative stages.
2. Separately describe the specific aspects of myorrhaphy of the levator muscles, reconstruction of the anal sphincter, or perineal repair in general.
3. Describe the different structures used during perineal reconstruction.

*S*ince Musset described this beautiful operation, the most recent modification has been the application of resorbable endo-anal sutures instead of non-resorbable material. Originally developed for the treatment of obstetrical perineal ruptures, its indications now also include the treatment of low recto-vaginal fistulas. The principle of this surgical intervention lies in re-establishing (1) the anal sphincter's continuity, where necessary, and (2) the normal length of the posterior vaginal wall by myorrhaphy of the anal levator ani and perineal superficial transversal muscles. Where the anal canal's length needs to be reconstructed due to an old rupture of obstetrical origin, or in the case of a low recto-vaginal fistula resulting from an earlier intervention, an anal suture is associated to this procedure.

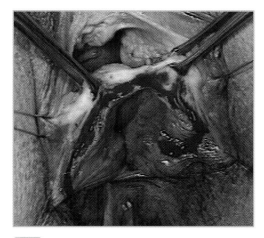

20.2 Initial incision with marking threads in place.

INDICATIONS

An old rupture of the anal sphincter and a recto-vaginal fistula of obstetrical origin, preceded by a primary section of the anal sphincter are the indications for this intervention.

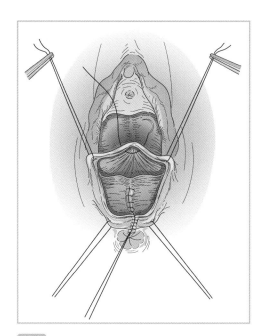

20.3 The anal canal has been sutured and the vaginal suture begins.

RELATED INTERVENTIONS

The following are related:
- anal sphincter repair following a complete perineal tear, complicated by vaginal birth;
- perineal reconstruction for vulvar malformations after obstetrical tear;
- myorrhaphy of the levator muscles.

DESCRIPTION

The described intervention is the repair of an old obstetrical tear, associating a perineal tear with that of the anal sphincter.

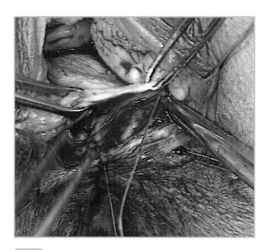

20.4 The anal sphincter's ends are taken up with a needle.

Positioning the Kocher forceps and marking threads

The old tear appears as a scarred transversal adhesion separating the ano-rectal and vaginal mucosa. The marking threads are placed at the level of the cutaneomucous delimitation, as well as at the vaginal position of the tear. The anal sphincter's ends are easily identified by an absence of an anal fold in concurrence with a small depression. A thread marks the bottom of the rupture on the side of the anal mucosa. The Kocher forceps are positioned at the level of the incision's cutaneous limits, but also across from the anal mucosa's limits and the perineal cutaneous edges.

Vaginal infiltration and vaginal and perineal incision

Once again, the recto-vaginal and sub-cutaneous dissection planes are prepared by vaginal infiltration at the level of the perineum. One can then carry out the incision by following the edges, vaginal mucosa then cutaneous mucosa, of the perineal tear before terminating at the level of the tear of the anal mucosa (figure 20.2).

Positioning the Allis' forceps

The Allis' forceps grasp the edges of the vaginal incision. They are then lifted in order to prepare the recto-vaginal dissection plane. Dissection of the recto-vaginal plane is performed using a cold scalpel and completed with scissors. This will enable mobilisation of the edges of the anal incision in order to reconstitute the anal canal.

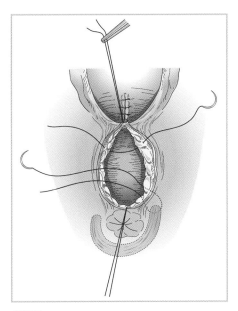

20.6 The vaginal suture is complete. The extremities of the sphincter are pulled together by performing a turning motion of the needle, without dissection the needle, without dissection.

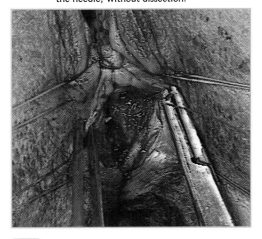

20.7 Union of the subcutaneous tissues.

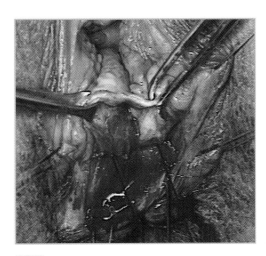

20.5 Low myorrhaphy.

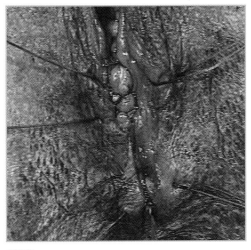

20.8 Final view.

Preparing the edges of the anal cicatrix and reconstituting the anal canal

The anal edges are freshened by closely cutting with scissors. The repair is carried out by bringing together (a) the edges of the cicatrix towards the limit of the tear with (b) the region of the cutaneo-mucous junction, by applying stitches that take hold of both the anal muscle and mucosa. The stitches are placed close to one another. The individual sutures are pulled tight before the next is placed. The last stitch is placed at the level of the anal border (*figures 20.3 and 20.4*).

Suture of the anal sphincter

The torn anal sphincter is now sutured. The sphincter's ends are identified at the level of the lateral depressions of retraction indicated above. A strong needle with a slowly resorbable suture is used to take hold of each the sphincter's ends, which are found towards the bottom and behind the radiating folds. By simple traction one verifies that the sphincter's end is firmly held, allowing it to be mobilised and put under tension. The two ends of the suture are now knotted on the midline (*figures 20.5 and 20.6*).

Myorrhaphy of the anal levator muscles

One can either perform a myorrhaphy of the low levator muscles underneath the posterior colporrhaphy or directly carry out the unification of the perineal muscles and of the subcutaneous tissues (*figure 20.7*).

Closure

The vaginal and, later, the perineal cutaneous closure is done with separate stitches using resorbable sutures (*figure 20.8*).

CHAPTER 21

Uterine preservation – Richardson operation

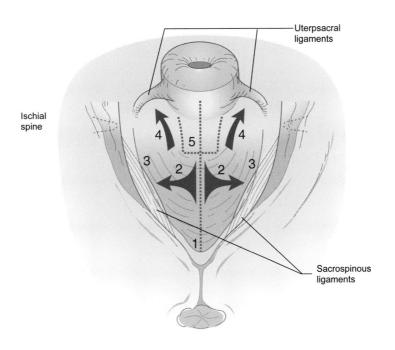

21.1 *Summary sketch.*
1. Incision. 2. Rectovaginal incision, opening of the pararectal foassae. 3. Dissection of the sacrospinous ligaments. 4. Dissection of the uterosacral ligaments. 5. Formation of the vaginal strips.

Guide to the reader

1. Determine the indications of this operation.
2. Recognise the common points with the Richter intervention.
3. Discuss the different techniques for uterine suspension to the sacrospinous ligaments.

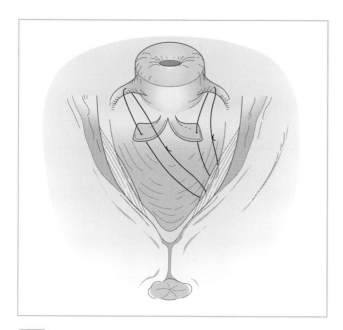

21.2 Scheme of the intervention.

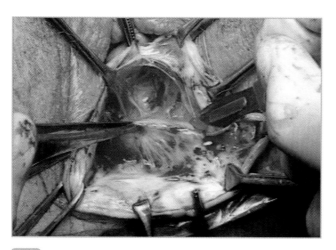

21.3 Rectal dissection.

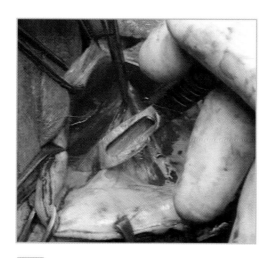

21.4 Low rectal dissection.

PRINCIPLE OF THE OPERATION

The Richardson operation consists of suspending the uterine isthmus and uterosacral ligaments to the sacrospinous ligament with a non-resorbable thread.

Although the procedure has several disadvantages, it also has one decisively important advantage: it offers the possibility for uterine suspension with conservation of the uterus via a vaginal approach, without affecting the patient's fertility and even permitting subsequent childbirth via the vaginal route.

The inconveniences are, firstly, linked to uterine conservation – the traction on the uterosacral ligaments draws the uterus into a posterior position – that could be the cause for secondary dyspareunias; and secondly, this intervention strongly resembles the direct uterine pexias with single-thread suspension of the uterine isthmus to the prevertebral ligament, which have been abandoned due to the frequency of redhibitory failure exceeding 50 %. This defect can be attenuated by associating operative procedures for prolapse treatment, such as that for cystocele, or with myorrhaphy of the levator muscles. However, these would diminish the possibility of subsequent childbirth via the vaginal route, which appears to us the sole indication for this intervention. Furthermore, the operation's success rate would in such a case be lower than that for abdominal intervention with uterine conservation. We prefer to apply the latter approach for patients under the age of 50.

INDICATIONS

Indications are rare:
- young patient;
- patient wishing to have children afterwards;
- patient unable to live with discomfort caused by a prolapse;
- patient with a predominant hysterocele;
- patient has been informed of the operations' temporary and incomplete nature;
- patient accepting the risk of relapse following childbirth.

If an older patient wishes to conserve her uterus, this technique will be associated to the other techniques that have already been described in relation with complete prolapse treatment. In this case, the Richardson intervention replaces the vaginal vault suspension according to Richter, from which it differs only in the suspension to the uterosacral ligaments. If required, it will be associated with cystocele treatment, if possible by the "plastron" technique. In addition, one will associate a myorrhaphy of the levator muscles with the procedure.

RELATED INTERVENTION

Suspension of the vaginal vault according to Richter (chapter 17) is technically very similar.

DESCRIPTION

The procedure consists of uterine suspension to the left sacrospinous ligament using two lengths of non-resorbable thread that are suspended to the uterosacral ligaments and to two vaginal strips fashioned at the level of the posterior vaginal pouch. Thus, the only difference to a Richter intervention lies in the suspension to the uterosacral ligaments; the aspect of uterine conservation does not modify the operative stages (*figure 21.2*).

Operational stages in common with Richter intervention

Since they have already been described in chapter 17, the following stages will not be detailed here:
– infiltration, vaginal incision of the total posterior wall and positioning of the Allis' forceps (*cf.* chapter 17);
– recto-vaginal dissection (*cf.* chapter 17) (*figures 21.3 and 21.4*);
– opening of the left pararectal fossa. We prefer to perform uterine suspension unilaterally, as explained in the chapter concerning the Richter suspension. As is true for the latter intervention, one must be able to perform a contralateral or bilateral suspension, should the ligament be of poor quality (*figure 21.5*);
– dissection of the sacrospinous ligament;
– passage of the needle through the ligament (*figure 21.6*);
– verification of the strength of the hold, and of homeostasis (*cf.* chapter 17).

Myorrhaphy of the levator muscles and verification of rectal integrity

If the patient wishes to subsequently give birth via the vaginal route, it is preferable to perform a partial procedure in order not to produce a contraindication to natural childbirth. Of course, absence of an associated myorrhaphy results in an elevated risk of secondary reoccurrence, especially of a rectocele.

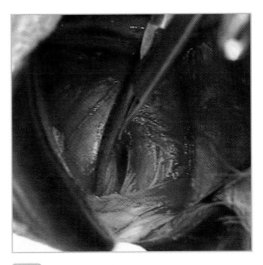

21.5 Opening the left pararectal fossa, the scissors distancing the levator muscles and rectum.

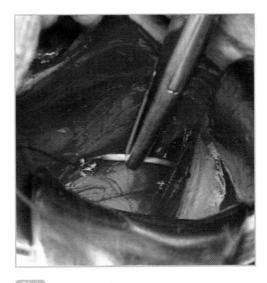

21.6 Thread inside the left sacrospinous ligament.

Uterine suspension

Before beginning with the vaginal closure, direct and indirect suspension of the uterus will be performed. Each non-resorbable thread that is passed through the left sacrospinous ligament is passed through one of the uterosacral ligaments. This passage must be solid in order to allow an efficient uterine suspension. However, it is not desirable to firmly bring the uterosacral and sacrospinous ligaments in contact with each other; this will only result in an excessive posterior tilt of the uterus. We prefer applying the procedure described in the chapter that treats the Richter intervention and produce two vaginal strips measuring about 2 cm by 3 cm for suspending the vaginal floor and supporting the suspension. Using this procedure there is no risk of obtaining an excessive uterine rotation, as only the vaginal strips will be brought into contact with the ligament.

Here, the choice for the vaginal strips' location is simplified by uterine conservation. Their bases should be positioned at the level of the posterior vaginal pouch. Each suspension thread is now passed through one of the vaginal strips and then through the homolateral uterosacral ligament (cf. figure 21.2).

Vaginal closure and putting the suspension threads under tension

Vaginal closure will commence at the level of the posterior pouch and then follow exactly the protocol described for the Richter intervention.

After having accomplished the vaginal closure and having verified homeostasis, one then counts the compresses.

CHAPTER 22

Uterine preservation – Manchester operation and Shirodkar technique

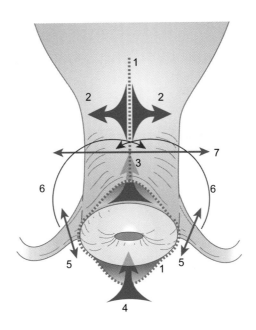

22.1 *Summary sketch.*
1. Percicervical vaginal "T" incision. 2. Dissection of the uterine isthmus. 3. Uterovesical dissection.
4. Posterior dissection. 5. Dissection and section of the sacrospinous ligaments. 6. Anterior crossing
of the utero-sacral ligaments. 7. Section of the cervix underneath the crossing.

Guide to the reader

1. Determine, in the series of operative stages, those steps that belong to the procedure for cervical amputation and those for the bringing of the utero-sacral ligaments under tension.
2. Give a detailed description of a treatment for cystocele.

The Manchester operation has been widely used with satisfactory results in the middle term. Its principle is based on the bringing under tension of the uterosacral ligaments that have been crossed and suspended to the uterine isthmus' anterior side (Shirodkar technique), in association with amputation of the uterine cervix. It thus has the advantage of conserving the patient's uterus while performing a uterine suspension technique using attached uterosacral ligaments brought back under tension (figure 22.2). Especially in the case of uterine elongation, frequently observed in conjunction with a hysterocele, this repositioning is made more efficient by amputating the uterine cervix. Although this procedure was originally proposed for the treatment of prolapse via a vaginal approach, it is also applied for treatment of cystocele and hysterocele. This intervention does not include any suspension technique, which has negative consequences for achieving long-lasting results. Furthermore, the indications are restricted to hysteroceles occurring in isolation, and the technique proves less successful in cases of associated cystocele. Furthermore, the frequent secondary appearance of urinary incontinence has been described.

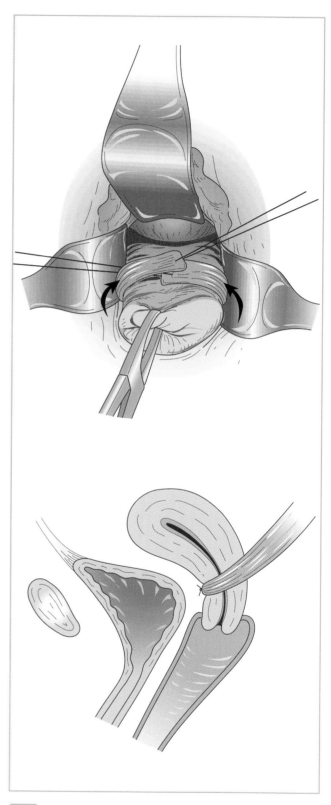

INDICATIONS

The only remaining indications are isolated hysteroceles in women desiring to keep their uterus; if a cystocele is associated, it must be moderate and not externalised.

INCONVENIENCES

They are numerous:
– impaired fertility by partial resection of the uterine cervix;
– risk of secondary cervical stenosis;
– shortening of the anterior vaginal wall;
– risk of a secondary rectocele.

RELATED INTERVENTIONS

The intervention has operative stages in common with:
– re-establishing tension of the uterosacral ligaments (Shirodkar technique);

22.2 Shirodkar technique.

– amputation of the uterine cervix or amputation using a cold scalpel for the Sturmdorf stitching technique used to cover the cervix with vaginal tissue.

DESCRIPTION

Positioning the Kocher forceps, infiltration

The operation begins with a "T" incision. One will thus start by positioning the Kocher forceps, then performing an infiltration as described for the paravaginal suspension. The Museux' forceps are placed on the uterine cervix and kept under traction.

"T" incision and positioning the Allis' forceps

The firm incision, as illustrated in the scheme, is performed using a cold scalpel and permits the positioning of the Allis' forceps onto the edges of the anterior and pericervical incisions. By spreading and lifting these forceps, the dissection planes will be made visible.

Vesicovaginal dissection

As for all interventions commencing with a "T" incision (paravaginal suspension, isolated Campbell's intervention), the incision is followed by a vesicovaginal dissection that allows the freeing of the anterior vaginal wall from its attachments in order to then be able to reposition the bladder. This dissection is laterally continued as far as the vaginal pouches, without opening the paravesical fossae (*figure 22.3*).

Uterovesical dissection

Because the uterus is to be conserved, the bladder's base at the uterus will be dissected in order to prepare the cervical amputation and to mobilise the bladder for its repositioning. This dissection is identical to that realised during vaginal hysterectomy without the necessity for an opening of the anterior pouch. The tissues stretched between the bladder and uterus are incised at the midpoint using scissors. The anterior retractor is now placed inside the space thus liberated, and the dissection is pursued beyond the uterine isthmus. A pericervical dissection will also be performed (*figure 22.4*).

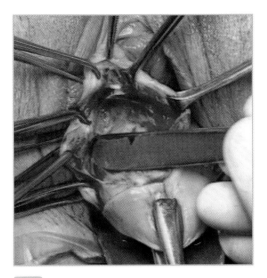

22.3 Anterior "T" incision, vesicovaginal dissection.

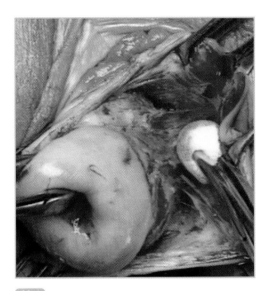

22.4 Pericervical dissection.

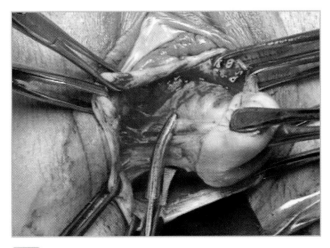

22.5 Grasping of the right uterosacral ligament.

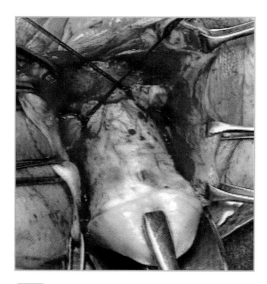

Anterior crossing of the two uterosacral
ligaments.

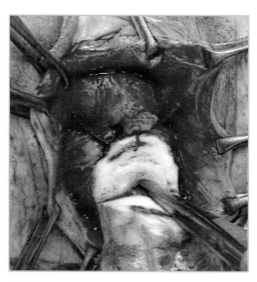

Following closure of the anterior colporrhaphy,
the cervix' anterior edge is sectioned.

Dissection of the uterosacral ligaments

The pericervical dissection, extended by an extensive dissection of the uterosacral ligaments, is performed as described for vaginal colpohysterectomy or Campbell's intervention (cf. chapter 14). It allows dissection of the posterior Douglas' pouch without opening it, as well as lateral dissection of the cervix and mobilisation of the pericervical vagina. As for this intervention, the uterosacral ligaments must be separated from the surrounding structures over an appropriate length that allows them to be crossed over the anterior side of the uterine isthmus.

Section of the uterosacral ligaments

Before dissecting the ligaments, it is often useful to section them at the point of contact at the uterine cervix. A Jean-Louis Faure forceps is easily placed perpendicular to and in close contact with the uterine cervix. One must ascertain that the hold on the ligament is sufficient and palpation with a finger before sectioning will assure that the posterior portion of the ligament is also well held (*figure 22.5*). It might sometimes be necessary to open the posterior pouch in order to facilitate a complete hold of these ligaments. The uterosacral ligament is ligatured with a thread and its dissection is then continued and facilitated by mobilising it with the help of a traction suture. Before terminating this operative stage, a simple simulation of the ligaments' mobility allows to ensure that the dissection performed effectively permits their crossing over the anterior side of the cervix.

Crossing of the uterosacral ligaments over the cervix and attachment to its anterior face

The uterosacral ligaments are pulled and brought onto the anterior portion of the uterine isthmus (*figure 22.6*). A non-resorbable thread is passed though the anterior wall of the isthmus. This will allow the usterosacral ligaments to be fixed in order to prevent their secondary displacement. A first ligament is fixed under tension; if necessary, the portion surpassing the isthmus will be resected. The second ligament is fixed using the same thread and the two ligaments are sutured to each other on the midline. If the uterine isthmus is now released, the uterine cervix will move upwards into place, as a consequence of the tension exerted on the uterosacral ligaments.

Closure of the anterior vaginal wall

The edges of the anterior incision can be sutured with a crossed overcast suture. Usually, a complementary bladder intervention is not associated. The continuous suture is terminated at the level of the uterine isthmus, across from the region of uterosacral ligament suspension.

Amputation of the uterine cervix

At this stage of the operation, the various dissections (peri-cervical, uterovesical, posterior, and that of the uterosacrals) will have resulted in the individualisation of the uterine cervix,

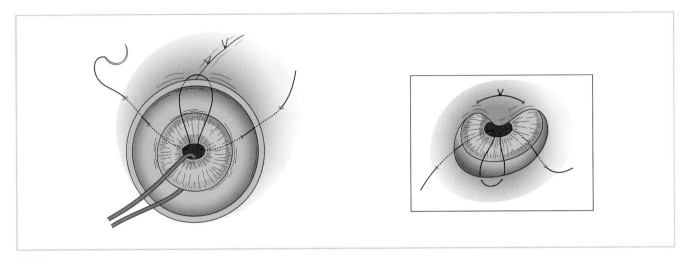

22.8   Sturmdorf stitch

which is free from its attachments to a point beyond the uterine isthmus, below the region where the uterosacral ligaments have been fixed. The uterosacral ligaments fixed on the isthmic anterior edge serve as a point of orientation for the section of the cervix, which begins at the anterior edge (*figure 22.7*). The incision's edges are grasped with two Pozzi's forceps that allow one to expose them without blocking the view. At this stage, the anterior Sturmdorf stitch is carried out (*figure 22.8*),before completing the posterior cervical section and, finally, performing the posterior closure stitch of Sturmdorf. This succession of events allows the cervix to remain under traction as long as possible without having to exert traction on the cervical stump, which would represent a risk for tearing and haemorrhage.

Before terminating the operation, the uterine cervix, and especially its section, must be covered for reasons of haemostasis and cervical surveillance without increasing the risk of a secondary stenosis. The cervical covering is done with Sturmdorf stitches in the front and back. At this stage of the procedure, there is often an excess of lateral vaginal tissue, which is resected, before laterally covering the section of the uterine cervix (*figure 22.9*).

After having verified haemostasis, the intervention ends with a count of the compresses.

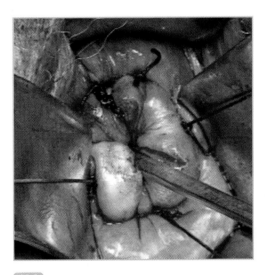

22.9   View at the end of the intervention.

CHAPTER 23

Recently developed techniques for the treatment of genital prolapse

Synthetic prostheses, and the transperineal and transobturator access routes

Guide to the reader

1. Discuss the interest of the novel techniques for prolapse treatment via a vaginal approach using synthetic prostheses.
2. Describe the anatomy and principle of the novel vaginal access routes described, namely transperineal and transobturator approaches, as well as the risks and the precautions that must be respected.

Numerous surgical techniques have been described for prolapse cures via a vaginal approach. Two main principles complement each other in relation to the techniques under evaluation. We shall first consider the use of supportive prostheses for prolapse treatment via a vaginal approach and then discuss two novel access routes for realising the suspensions via the vagina.

USAGE OF PROSTHESES VIA A VAGINAL APPROACH

There are many arguments in favour of using protheses via a vaginal approach during prolapse treatment. Without going into too much detail, the main arguments are the support provided and the availability of excessive tissue required for extended repair. Further incentives are the limits faced by today's techniques using biological materials with variable stability, the restrictive indications of techniques based on the enclosure of vaginal tissue, the extent of available vaginal tissue, the cases of pre-menopausal patients, and, finally, the considerable frequency of relapse seen with techniques using supports of tissue-origin. However, those who have tried to use synthetic protheses for the treatment of urinary incontinence are, unfortunately, aware of the potential complications, which include granulomas, slowness of healing, and secondary resections depending on the type of technique applied and the material used.

The application of prostheses via a vaginal approach a priori brings with it an elevated risk of complications, related to the amount of material required, to the proximity of the vaginal sutures, and to the sometimes poor quality of the vaginal tissue that covers them.

Theoretically, the ideal solution would have been the use of resorbable prostheses that disappear following the formation of a healing fibrosis sufficient to maintain the anatomical result of the intervention. Unfortunately, animal experiments and even experimental applications in humans have not been able to validate such an approach, since the tissues' resorption times were too short to obtain satisfactory results.

In a parallel development, there has been progress in the preparation and purification of these prosthesis, including the application of Prolene. The better tolerance of these synthetic materials favour their increased use.

If one decides to use synthetic tissues, one has the choice between several application principles:

– the first is simply to support the vaginal cicatrices by placing a synthetic tissue beneath the anterior and posterior vaginal colporraphies. This technique, not particularly logical, is neither based on clinical observations (the relapses observed are not at the level of the vaginal cicatrices) nor on a biomechanical understanding.

– a second approach is to apply the prostheses directly as a support between the viscera, over their total surface, and the vaginal tissue. In this case, the prosthesis is suspended underneath a viscera. One can thus realise a plastron identical to the description given earlier, but substituting the synthetic tissue for vaginal tissue. In such a case, the dissections will be as extensive as for the classical techniques, and the same procedure for suspending the threads by passing the needle through the ligaments will be applied. The technical description will vary only concerning the vaginal incision and the vaginal conservation. It is equally possible to place a posterior prosthesis suspended bilaterally to the sacrospinous ligaments as done during Richter's intervention; the risk of the prosthesis performing a secondary retro-action, which would result in the tearing away of the suspension points, reduces the interest in these techniques;

– the third application mode is based on the principle of the "tension-free" urinary incontinence treatment. Here, the above described tissue reinforcement is accompanied by a threadless suspension using a synthetic strip that remains inside the tissues and the aponeurosis. This approach, which simplifies positioning of the prostheses, is poorly described as "tension-free", since there is a very real tension that must be adjusted according to the desired anatomical outcome. The term "prosthesis without suspension" appears to be more precise, since there is no suspension thread to hold the prosthesis in place, which could eventually retract secondarily.

DESCRIPTION OF NOVEL ACCESS ROUTES

These techniques concern the suspensions to the sacrospinous ligament, as well as those to the pelvic fascia's tendinous arches. These should not be considered as techniques in their own right, but rather as novel access routes to these ligaments that allow application of the suspension methods. After having described the anatomical principle and surgical basis that have led to the development of the new access routes, we will consider the suspensions possible using threads or the popular "tension-free" suspensions.

These two techniques have been developed in order to place prostheses without tension, putting in place in the front an equivalent to a suspension to the tendinous arches and in the back an equivalent to a suspension to the sacrospinous ligament. In fact, their suspension principles are not comparable.

The transobturator suspension is based on blocking the

prosthesis inside the middle pelvic aponeurosis, which, though often thin and of variable stability, is sufficient if a wide prosthesis is being placed. Its application in cystocele treatment has been developed by Bernard Jacquetin. In von Theobald's technique, the posterior suspension does not rely on a suspension to the ligament or to the aponeurosis, but on a blocking effect, obtained mainly by use of the levator muscles. For those using this latter technique, it represents a valid alternative to Richter' suspension, although in reality it is comparable to a suspension to a high myorrhaphy. The exit position of the needle, as well as the amount of levator muscle taken hold of, is decided by the surgeon. The resistance appears to depend on the height of the placement and on the quality of the levator muscles.

Here, we will describe a variant using positioning via a trans-perineal approach. Readapting the principle of suspension to the sacrospinous ligament with a retro-passage of the needle through the ligament, this alternative technique also makes use of a trans-perineal approach. However, this technique appears to guarantee a suspension that is of higher quality, more solid, and anatomically better positioned. As in the case for the transobturator prosthesis, one uses two arms that are passed behind the sacrospinous ligaments that are left without suspension, blocked by the ligaments.

Suspension to the pelvic fascia's tendinous arches via a transobturator approach, a rather seductive approach, has been described for surgical treatment of urinary incontinence (cf. chapter 26). Based on the passage of a needle, originating from the obturator orifice, through the pelvic aponeurosis, this technique allows either (1) the implementation of a suspension effect to the pelvic fascia's tendinous arches by suspending a thread to the middle aponeurosis, or (2) the placement of a "tension-free" prosthesis, blocked inside the middle pelvic aponeurosis.

In order to be complete, this suspension must be achieved with two arms on either side, as described by B. Jacquetin. The first arm is placed nearly retro-pubally, while the second passes 1 cm in front of the ischial spine through the tendinous arch.

TECHNIQUES

Cystocele treatment by placement of a subvesical prosthesis via a transobturator approach

Since the preparatory stages are similar to those performed for other techniques of cystocele treatment, we will not describe them here in detail, referring the reader instead to the corresponding chapters. Specifically, for the incision stages, please refer to the description of paravaginal suspension, and for the dissection stages, see the stages up to the opening of the paravesical fossae. If a vaginal hysterectomy is associated, we prefer to carry this out at the beginning of the procedure,

as is also done in the case of other cystocele treatments. Vesical dissection must be extensive in order to enable the prosthesis' positioning; the prosthesis itself should be broad and remain mobile after positioning in order to take into account the phenomenon of secondary retraction.

Placing the Kocher forceps, infiltration, incision

These stages resemble those realised during cystocele cure with a plastron, with the exception that the initial incision will in this case be median.

Vesico-vaginal dissection, opening the paravesical fossae

The bladder's lateral dissection is identical, but the opening of the paravesical fossae is more restricted, providing just enough space to allow the surgeon's finger to pass through. At this stage of the operation, the obturator orifice can be palpated with a finger inserted into the paravesical fossa; the needle can then be giuided by the finger once it has been passed, thus protecting the bladder from possible injury.

Cutaneous incision opposite the obturator orifice

For the placement of a sub-vesical prosthesis, the incision line will lie below the obturator orifice, 2 cm outside the urethral orifice. This incision should be about 3 mm in length to allow the needle's passage, positioned in the inguinal fold. The pre-spinal arm is put into place by a more lateral incision of about 1 cm, located about 2 cm lower, offering passage to the lower part of the obturator orifice.

The needle's passage under control of the finger

The needle must possess a strong, hooked curvature, since it must follow the anatomy of the obturator orifice, without having the handle jamming against the lower thigh (figure 23.1).

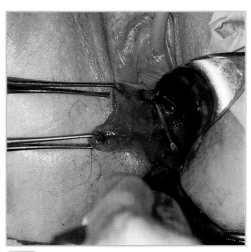

23.1 Transobturator passage of the needle.

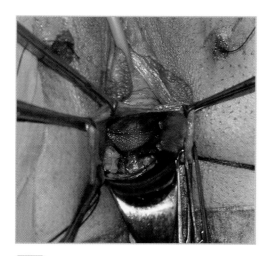

23.2 Anterior prosthesis in place.

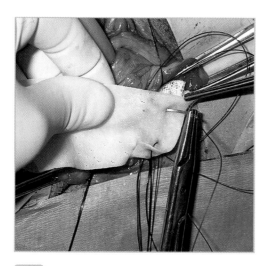

23.3 Pelvicol.

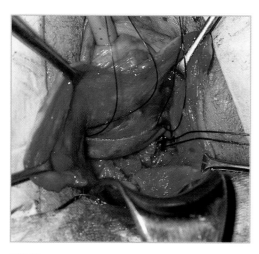

23.4 Pelvicol in place beneath the bladder.

Placing the thread or prosthesis inside the needle

The prosthesis' arm, or a thread that is fixed to the prosthesis, is passed through the needle's eye.

Adjusting the tension

For the anterior prosthesis, adjustment of the tension will be easy, since at maximal tension the prosthesis will end up a the level of the pelvic fascia's tendinous arches, an anatomically favourable position. However, given the secondary retraction phenomenon, we prefer to leave the prosthesis floating below the bladder in order to avoid secondary lateral slipping (figure 23.2).

Positioning the anterior prosthesis

The prosthesis' arms having been blocked laterally, it is unrolled underneath the bladder. The vagina is then closed with a continuous overcast suture without resection. In the case of an associated vaginal floor suspension, the posterior suspension will put the anterior wall back under tension. If this technique is used to treat an isolated cystocele, the vaginal floor must be fixed to the prosthesis, using at least a resorbable thread, which would allow it to remain in contact with the prosthesis after healing.

Cystocele cure by suspension of a synthetic plastron to the pelvic fascia's tendinous arches

This is exactly the same technique as the plastron technique with a median incision. Dissection of the bladder and opening of the paravesical trenches are identical. The transobturator passage is performed exactly as described above. It is advisable to take the same precaution not to apply any tension in order to prevent a secondary retraction (figures 23.3 and 23.4).

Suspension to the sacrospinous ligament via a trans-perineal approach

This technique, described by Papapetros and simplified by von Theobald, is proposed for the treatment of vaginal-vault prolapses. The trans-perineal approach is very seductive, due to the easy access it provides and its relative safety.

The suspension is effectuated using a tension-free, transperineal, trans-levator strip: posterior IVS in von Theobald's description.

In our view, its main drawback is the poor lateral hold provided by the prosthesis' arms passed inside the levator muscle. Here, there is no aponeurotic passage, which, though facilitating the prosthesis' positioning, is the reason for its fragility in case of an atrophic muscle, which occurs quite frequently. In any case, the strip is placed in a plane that lies above that of the sacrospinous ligament, but also closer to the surgeon. Suspension is performed on the prosthesis' median part, lying even higher up, so as not to compress the rectum. The position resembles that of a posterior ligamentopexy in axial terms, but is overall lower. Furthermore, the strip (IVS) can allow a vaginal vault suspension by use of a suspension stitch, but does not cover the rectum, meaning that another prosthesis would have to be attached.

This technique uses a trans-perineal approach, except for the bilateral placement of the posterior prosthesis' arms inside the sacrospinous ligament. The result is a bilateral suspension equivalent to that used for a cystocele treatment via a transobturator approach.

The first four stages are exactly the same as during a vaginal vault suspension according to Richter:
– posterior incision following positioning of the Kocher forceps and infiltration;
– recto-vaginal dissection;
– opening of the two pararectal fossae;
– dissection of the two sacrospinous ligaments.
Followed by (*figure 23.5*):
– bilateral perineal incision
– two 3 mm incisions on both sides of the midline, 3 cm laterally, and 3 cm below the anus;
– passage of the needle: positioned as for the IVS technique, the needle is passed laterally along the rectum under control of a finger before exiting laterally through the levator muscle. Here, the needle is less bent than that used during a transobturator approach. One can now easily take hold of the sacrospinous ligament with the needle that is now in the field of view (figure 23.6);
– putting the prosthesis into place: the prosthesis' arms are passed through the needle's eye on either side. The tension is adjusted at the end of the procedure (*figure 23.7*);
– the vaginal floor is fixed to the prosthesis' arms in order to obtain its bilateral suspension.

Attaching the vaginal floor via a "posterior" transobturator approach

This technique, described by Mellier, is based on the same principles as the posterior IVS technique; passage of the synthetic strip via a transobturator approach is extremely seductive for anatomical reasons, reducing the risk of injury to the rectum and carrying out a suspension along the vagina's axis.

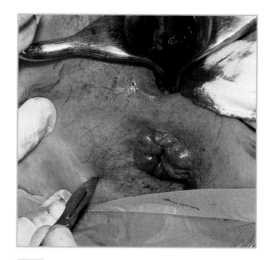

23.5 Perineal incisions.

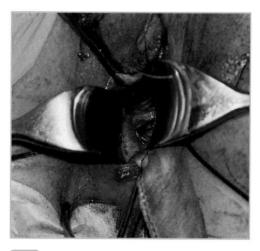

23.6 Trans-perineal needle passed inside the sacrospinous ligament.

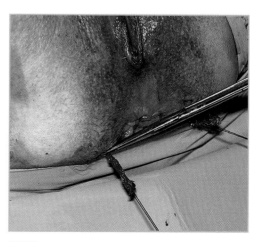

23.7 Posterior prosthesis, its arms exiting at the level of the perineum.

The intervention's description includes many operational stages that have already been described:

– posterior incision following positioning of the Kocher forceps and infiltration;

– rectovaginal dissection;

– opening of the two pararectal spaces, without dissection of the sacrospinous ligaments, but allowing the positioning of a retractor that pushed back the rectum during the needle's exit;

– incision opposite the obturator's orifice: for a sub-vesical prosthesis the incision will be located on the obturator orifice's lower part, 2 cm outside the urethral orifice. This incision should be about 3 mm long in order to allow passage of the needle;

– passage of the needle: positioned as for incontinence or cystocele treatment via a transobturator approach, the needle is passed laterally along the rectum under control of a finger before exiting laterally through the levator muscle.

– placing of the prosthesis: the prosthesis' arms are passed through the needle's eye on either side. The tension is adjusted at the end of the intervention, after having fixed the prosthesis to the vaginal vault.

Complete prolapse treatment according to the prosthetic TVM technique

This technique has been developed by a team of 9 gynaecological surgeons under the friendly encouragement of Bernard Jacquetin. This group includes Claude Rosenthal, Richard Villet, Georges Eglin, Juan Berrocal, Philippe Debodinance, Philippe Mage, Henri Clavé and Michel Cosson.

This original technique is still being evaluated, but appears promising. Here, we will reproduce the simplified description as given by Bernard Jacquetin, as well as the technical schemes for which we have been authorised by the authors and the Gynecare laboratory that has sponsored this group.

It consists in the placement of a synthetic prosthesis made of soft prolene:

– anterior inter-vesicovaginal prosthesis inserted like a hammock underneath the bladder, lying laterally against the ATFP (arcus tendinous fascia pelvis), held in place by two bilateral transobturator arms that are not fixed (figure 23.8):

– anteriorly, 1-2 cm from the ATFP's proximal (pre-pubic) region,

– posteriorly, 1-2 cm from the ATFP's distal (pre-spinal) region.

– posterior inter-rectovaginal prosthesis inserted in front of the rectum and lying laterally against the anal levator muscles, held in place by a lateral arm that is fixed bilaterally to or passing through the sacrospinous ligament's median part and fixed onto the tendinous centre of the perineum via its trans-perineal elongation.

This prosthesis can be used as a continuous or discontinuous prosthesis (after sectioning the intermediate portion if the prosthesis comes in a single piece procedure).

Principles of the intervention

Hysterectomy

Hysterectomy is systematically performed according to the technique described earlier in this work should the patient not have undergone such a procedure at an earlier date. Nevertheless, a peritonisation will be carried out in order to separate the prosthesis from the peritoneal cavity.

Anterior stage

This is closely related to that described for cystocele treatment. The result obtained by placing this anterior prosthesis is illustrated in figure 23.8.

The vagina will be closed sagittally, without colpectomy or after a simple refreshening of the edges should the vaginal section have been performed with an electrical scalpel. A resorbable, ideally Monocryl single-strand, thread will be used for the vaginal suture, applied in a simple, passed, or inverted overcast suture.

Median stage

If using a single-piece prosthesis, the uterosacral ligaments will have to be attached in front of the prosthesis, opposite its intermediate portion. The same can be done with the cardinal ligament and utero-adnexal ligaments, but this is not absolutely necessary.

If the prostheses are independent, the anterior prosthesis can remain free, pushed underneath the bladder and attached to the parametrium or uterosacral ligament. The posterior prosthesis can also remain free, simply pushed opposite from the Douglas' pouch or attached to the uterosacral ligaments or to the vaginal angles of the hysterectomy section.

In a hysterectomy has previously been carried out, there is often no identifiable structure. If the uterosacral ligaments still exist, they can be used in the same way. Otherwise, the intermediate portion of a continuous prosthesis will not be fixed.

Posterior stage

It is identical to the technique described for a suspension to the sacrospinous ligament via a trans-perineal approach.

The rectovaginal dissection will be carried out as usual, up to the opening of the pararectal fossa. The rectum will be lowered to the sacrum's lateral border, and the sacrospinous ligament can be identified by palpation all the way from its insertion at the level of the sacrum to its end at the level of the ischial spine. The technique is exactly the same as for the sacrospinofixation according to Richter.

A Monocryl suture can be used to carry out a plicature of the pre-rectal fascia.

The prosthesis' arms are either fixed trans-ligamentally, as previously described (figure 23.9), or directly at the level of the sacrospinous ligament's median part (figure 23.10), using a threaded needle or an instrument (including an Endostitch), using a non-resorbable thread that is fixed to the posterior prosthesis' C-branch.

The prosthesis is then spread out by 1 to 2 complementary threads that can be positioned bilaterally over the anal levator muscles, at the prosthesis' outer edge, in order to obtain a better positioning; and then on the lower part onto the perineal tendinous centre by applying one or more Vicryl stitches, depending on whether a perineorrhaphy is associated or not. The goal is to enclose this perineal elongation and to prevent or treat the syndrome of descending perineum.

As for the anterior stage, the vagina will be closed without colpectomy or after a simple refreshening of the edges should the vaginal section have been performed with an electrical scalpel. Closure of the posterior vaginal wall is carried out with a simple, passed or inverted overcast suture.

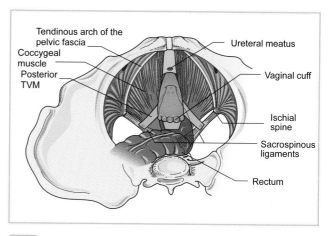

23.9 Prerectal prosthesis fixed to the sacrospinous ligaments.

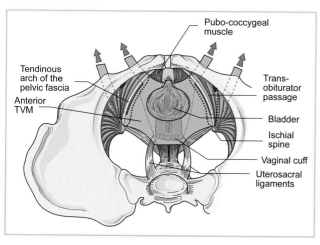

23.8 Subvesical transobiturator prosthesis.

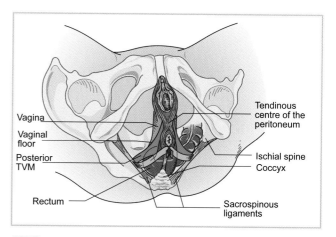

23.10 Prerectal trans-ligamental prosthesis.

Urinary incontinence

PART 6

Urinary incontinence: generalities

The objectives of this part are to:
-- describe the main vaginal surgical interventions for the treatment of urinary incontinence;
-- list their respective advantages and disadvantages;
-- identify the operational stages they have in common, as well as the specificities of each procedure;
-- be able to describe the techniques for accessing the Retzius space in detail;
-- comment on the procedures for preventing bladder injury, the signs pointing towards such a complication, and the techniques used for treating it.

Over the past few years, the treatment of urinary incontinence has been subject to important technical changes, mainly due to the introduction of sub-urethral sling techniques, in particular of TVT (Tension-free Vaginal Tape) (figure 1).

As a result of a number or randomised studies, Marion-Kelly type anterior colporrhaphy techniques, as well as indirect suspension techniques, such as those of Raz, Pereyra, Stamey or others, which we will not describe here, have been gradually abandoned over the past few years (figure 2).

The two techniques that are still being performed are the colposuspensions according to Burch and the sling technique with placement at the level of the urethro-vesical junction using mixed access routes (figure 3).

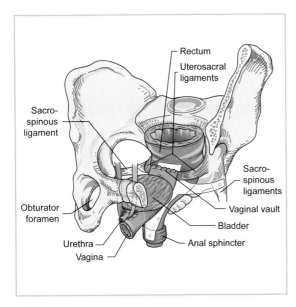

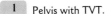

1 Pelvis with TVT.

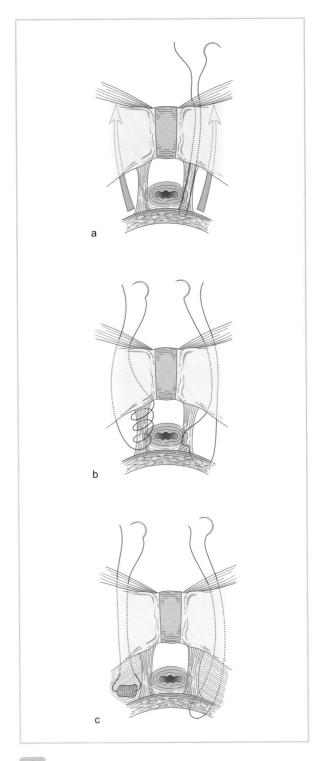

2 Different suspension techniques.
a) schematic views of the principle, showing the analogy between a retropubic colpopexy operation on the left and an operation using mixed access routes on the right.
b) Pereyra operation on the left, Raz operation on the right.
c) Stamey operation on the left, Gittes operation on the right.

Following the phenomenal success of the sub-urethral "TVT" sling, numerous techniques making use of sub-urethral slings have evolved. We will not describe all of these techniques in detail, but will focus on those representing an innovation or, above all, a simplification of the technique. We will also present the sling technique as described by Crépin, which uses vaginal tissue. Although not a procedure for the treatment of isolated incontinence, it may represent an interesting and economical alternative, especially in cases of urinary incontinence associated to a genital prolapse in menopausal patients.

The indications are urinary incontinence:
- that is stress induced;
- having been confirmed during a clinical examination using a stress test and/or during a urodynamic evaluation;
- lowering the quality of life;
- sometimes hidden by an associated genital prolapse.

Since Ulmsten's original description, the techniques for the treatment of urinary incontinence have undergone many modifications. Thus, some surgeons do not place an intravesical support to tip the bladder away from the needle's passage. Many do not perform a cystoscopy after each passage of the needle, while others position the prosthesis without regulating its tension according to the patient's urinary leakages. None of these modifications have been scientifically validated. They cannot be recommended for surgeons in training, since only experience will allow some of these precautions to be omitted.

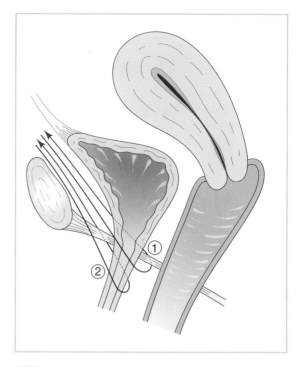

3 Classic sling (I). TVT, tension-free vaginal tape (2).

CHAPTER 24

Suburethral slings

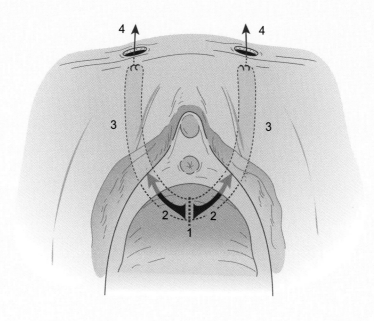

24.1 *Summary sketch.*
1. 1-cm incision opposite the urethra's middle third. 2. Lateral dissection. 3. Passage of the needle. 4. Adjustment of tension.

Guide to the reader

1. Indicate the physiopathological hypotheses explaining the efficiency of the suburethral slings, as well as their indications.
2. Precisely detail the stages for placement of the slings.
3. Describe the risks existing during and after these operations and the precautions to be taken to avoid them.
4. Discuss the advantages and disadvantages of each suburethral slings.

*W*ithin few years, the synthetic suburethral slings have, in France, become the model intervention for the treatment of stress-induced urinary incontinence. This rapid change might appear excessive, considering that the long-term evaluations have not yet been completed. Nevertheless, simplicity of the technique together with excellent functional short-term results and a low frequency of complications explain at least partially this trend. The success has given rise to copy with or without technical advantages, which we will discuss in this chapter's second part.

INDICATIONS

The synthetic suburethral slings are indicated:
– in case of stress-induced urinary incontinence;
– if urinary incontinence has been confirmed by clinical examination, with a stress test and/or during an urodynamic check-up;
– if urinary incontinence diminishes the quality of life;
– if urinary incontinence is hidden by an associated genital prolapse;
– in case of a positive result for the TVT-test or Ulmsten test.

RELATED TECHNIQUES

The pathway through the Retzius space is identical to that realised during interventions for "classical" slings.

THE TVT STRIP

As Honour is to be given where it is due, we will provide a detailed description of the first strip, commercialised under the name Tension-free Vaginal Tape (TVT).

The technique described here is inspired by the original procedure, but includes some minor changes for the sake of simplification. It is performed under local anaesthesia accompanied by intravenous administration of an analgesic drug, or under loco-regional rachianesthesia after informed consent of the patient.

Installation, infiltration

The patient is installed in a gynaecological position, but avoiding the bending of the thighs too far back, which, although facilitating access to the vagina, reduces the needle's exit space by bringing the large blood vessels towards each other. The bladder is emptied and we perform a local anaesthesia by infiltrating a 1:2 mixture of adrenaline-containing Xylocaïne and physiological serum: 60 ml are infiltrated via a sub-pubic approach on either side into the Retzius space. 20 ml are administered retropubally on either side, and about 10 ml are injected under the vaginal incision.

This infiltration results in local anaesthesia, and further has the advantage of distancing the bladder due to an increased volume of the surrounding tissue. Even if the intervention is carried out under loco-regional anaesthesia, we always carry out this infiltration. Two Kocher forceps are positioned in order to mark and display the incision's path. The first forceps is placed about 2 cm from the urethral orifice.

Preparation of the equipment and emptying of the bladder

While waiting for the local anaesthesia to take effect, the material is prepared by positioning the first needle to the handle. Before beginning the procedure, the bladder is completely emptied. Apparently, attempting to position the bladder is not indispensable during needle passage, infiltration of the Retzius space being the best security measure for the prevention of a transvesical path.

Incision

One performs an incision of about 1 cm length opposite the urethra's middle third, which is identified and exposed by two Kocher forceps that pull along the vaginal path (*figure*

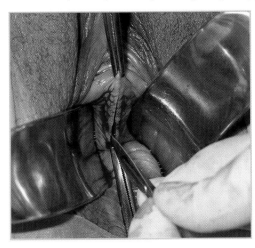

24.2 Vaginal incision opposite the urethra's middle third.

24.2). The urethra having been distanced by the infiltration, this incision must be firm, sectioning the entire vaginal wall in one go.

Vaginal dissection

The incision's edges are gripped with an Allis' forceps on either side and the Kocher forceps, which are useless at this stage, are removed. Traction is applied to the forceps in order to create an entry space for the small dissection scissors. The scissors are oriented towards the pubic symphysis and pushed as far as the sub-symphyseal space, verifying with a finger that the vaginal pouch is not perforated (*figure 24.3*). It is not necessary to dissect any further, and the scissors are now opened about 1 cm wide, all the while keeping them within the sub-symphyseal space. The opened scissors are pulled outwards, which enlarges the original dissection path and prepares the needles' passage.

Passage of the needle

One can now position the TVT needles. Traction is again applied to the Allis' forceps and the needle is inserted, on the side one has chosen to commence with, as far as the previously dissected sub-symphyseal space. During this positioning procedure, the needle is oriented along the previously dissected path and oriented laterally without effort (*figure 24.4*). The Allis' forceps are now released and, gripping the needle's end, the needle's point is reoriented towards the midline, targeting the infiltration about 1 cm from the midline, above the pubis (*figure 24.5*). The skin can be breached without a scalpel incision and the needle is left in place. The same action is performed contralaterally.

Bladder injury, cystoscopy
In case of bladder injury, we proceed as follows :
– removal of the needle, emptying of the bladder, repositioning the needle now avoiding the perforation zone, cystoscopic examination;
– maintenance of a catheter for 24 hours and monitoring of the mictions and post-mictional residues after its removal.
In case of repeated urinary injury:
– one must verify vesical integrity by cystoscopy upon the needle's new passage;
– problems of adjustment might be encountered due to urinary leakages, located at the level of the vagina along the path of the needle's passage, occurring during coughing stress; – the catheter is maintained for 24 hours.

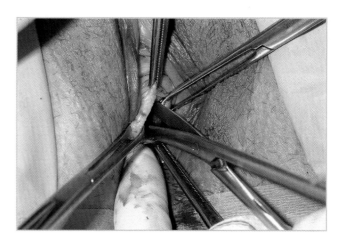
24.3 Lateral dissection.

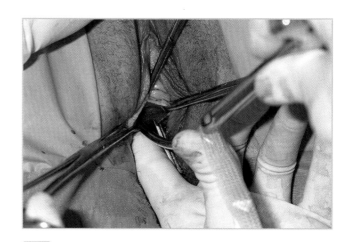
24.4 Positioning the needle via a vaginal approach.

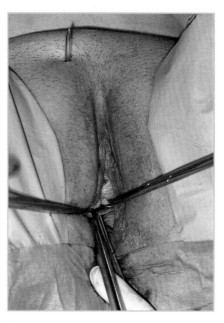
24.5 Exit of the needles above the pubis.

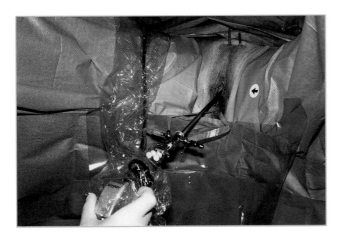

24.6 Cystoscopy.

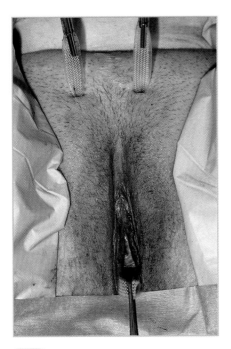

24.7 View of the prosthesis in place.

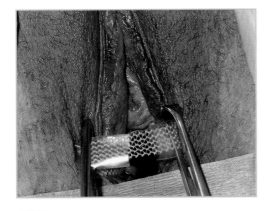

24.8 Partial removal of the strip hemi-sheaths.

Cystoscopy

Once the thread has been passed on either side without yet having inserted the strip into the tissue, a cystoscopic exam is performed (*figure 24.6*). The presence of a needle inside the bladder requires its removal and repositioning once the bladder has been emptied. It is not always easy to visualise a transfixing needle during the course of the cystoscopy. In fact, the needle's silvery colour is sometimes confused with the reflection of the bubbles that are often present in front of the anterior vesical wall. Furthermore, locating the bladder's injuries, which are in the majority of cases proximal to the midline and very close to the pubic symphysis, is not always easy without articulated optical mounts. It may occur that the bladder injury is not identified during cystoscopy, and that a small flow of urine is observed along the sheaths of the strips after the needle has been removed. In such a case, another device must be put in place, since the needle cannot be removed via the same route.

Putting the strip into place

After having assured a correct placement of the threads, the prosthesis is positioned sub-urethrally by pulling on the threads, leaving the sheaths in place (*figure 24.7*). During this same stage, one will also exert a moderate traction via the vaginal approach on the ends of the sheath that cross at the midline. The goal of this traction is to reduce the spanning tension so that the ablation of the sheaths can be performed with reduced traction during the following step (figure 24.8).

An Allis' forceps is positioned spanning the prosthesis and its sheath, allowing a contra-traction to be exerted in case an excessive tension is applied.

In case of haemorrhage during the operation

The risk of damaging a large blood vessel is very low, below 1/1000, and is linked to incorrect positioning of the needles: overly lateral passage of the needle, patient's thighs too folded. Emergency laparotomy is required.

More typically, the haemorrhage originates from a blood vessel of the Retzius space which does not permit haemostasis. If the bleeding persists after having placed the strip and adjusted the tension, an intravaginal gauze pad is put into place and the catheter is clamped for two hours with 200 cm3 inside the bladder.

Adjusting the tension during coughing

The strip's tension is regulated after having filled the bladder with 250 ml of physiologic serum. An experienced surgeon can regulate the tension under general anaesthesia without a coughing test. However, in most cases this adjustment results in good efficiency and avoids excessive tension. As for the Ulmsten technique, one should ideally adjust for a slight urinary leakage and, above all, avoid over-adjusting (*figure 24.10*).

Once the adjustment has been made, the two protective sheaths are removed. In order to do this, the prosthesis has to be blocked into place sub-urethrally by using the Allis forceps still in position; this is done to avoid additional tension that can be created by rubbing during the removal of the sheaths.

After removal of the sheaths, one verifies that the applied tension corrects urinary leakage while allowing minimal leakages to persist.

Acute urinary retention

Rare, representing less than 1 % of the cases, this results from excessive tension of the strip: one must follow the guideline of minimal urinary leakage. Most often, the condition is linked to a hypotonic bladder or from a pre-operative mictional residue: in such a case, the patient must be informed.

In the case of complete retention: a secondary section of the prosthesis is carried out sub-urethrally before d8. This section is performed under loco-regional or local anaesthesia and is accompanied by: reopening of the vaginal incision, palpating the sub-urethral prosthesis with a finger, cutting with a cold scalpel without opening the urethra, which has been mobilised with a metal bougie and lowered after traction.

By the same technique one can perform a simple "release" of the strip, placing closed scissors between urethra and strip by pressing down hard.

In the case of incomplete retention (residue superior to 100 cm^3), self-catheterisation will be performed three times a day until return to normal.

Section of the strip

Once the adjustment has been performed, the strip is sectioned above the pubis at skin level so that the strip can retract from the cutaneous plane (*figure 24.11*). After having realised this section, traction is applied to the skin with forceps to free the skin's deeper layers, thus ensuring the retraction (*figure 24.12*).

Control of haemostasis

Haemostasis is verified after adjusting the strip. Persistent bleeding might require the putting into place of a vaginal gauze pad and catheter for 24 hours.

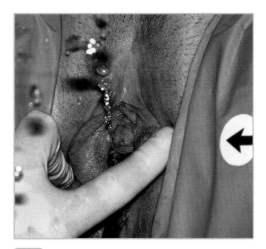
24.9 Urinary leakage during adjustment.

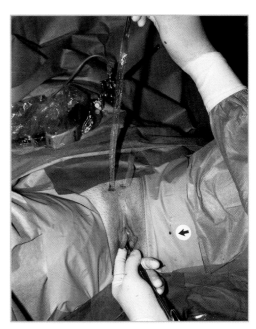
24.10 Blocking the prosthesis while removing the supporting sheaths.

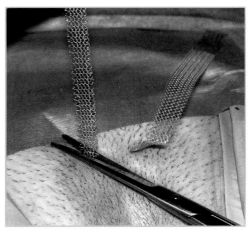
24.11 Section of the strip above the pubis.

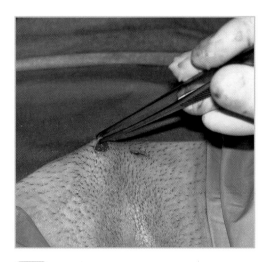

24.12 Traction on the skin in order to distance the prosthesis before closure.

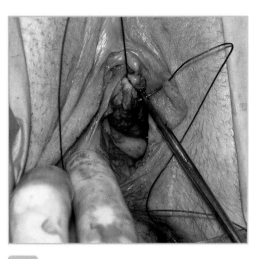

24.13 Vaginal closure.

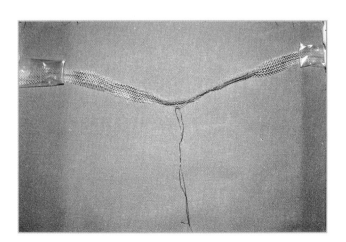

24.14 AMS strip.

Vaginal closure by crossed overcast suture

The vagina is closed using a no. 1 resorbable thread (*figure 24.13*).

In case of secondary intolerance to the strip
False intolerance occurs in the case of a transfixing passage at the level of the vaginal pouch while positioning the needle.

The true intolerance (rare, about 1 %) requires resection by the vaginal approach of the externalised element of the prosthesis, with: traction on the prosthesis, then lateral vaginal dissection and resection of the prosthesis' visible portion; then vaginal closing by a couple of resorbable stitches.

Closure of cutaneous counter-incisions

Finally, the cutaneous plane will be closed with a single stitch of high-resorption thread at the position of each of the cutaneous counter-incisions.

Section of the strip near the skin
Careful: if the prosthesis is left too close in contact with the skin, there is a risk of granuloma formation with fibres surpassing the skin.

Prevention: traction is applied during sectioning of the strip, followed by cutaneous mobilisation.

OTHER SUB-URETHRAL STRIPS

We will merely discuss those products that represent an innovation or technical simplification deserving to be described, and ask the readers to contact the various companies for more detailed information on these products:

-- prosthesis-variation: only one of the products is made of silicon-sheathed polyester in order to reduce the risk of an intolerance towards the prosthesis (one of the two *Lift* strips);

-- variation in accessing the Retzius space: surgeons experienced in suspension techniques using a needle sometimes prefer to position the strip from top to bottom, passing through the Retzius space;

-- variation in access route: transobturator approach; for the time being, this extremely seductive way of positioning the strip is only possible with products from the Porges laboratory or with the *Lift*.

Some technical details have also evolved. Thus, the prosthesis' sheath is not always necessary. Some prosthesis slide into place without the requirement of a secondary mobilisation, thus simplifying the procedure. In fact, the absence of a protective sheathing does not appear to have any implications on secondary infections of the strip; the rarely occurring infections seem rather to correlate with the limited contact of the prosthesis with the vagina.

Several products, e.g. the *IVS* bandage from Tyco or that from AMS, make use of needles onto or into which the adaptors that hold the prosthesis are placed, which requires additional manipulation.

The latter has an incorporated thread that facilitates counter-traction in case when excessive tension has been applied (*figures 24.14 and 24.15*); its removal is performed after having adjusted the tension.

In the following part of this chapter we will describe the *Lift* procedure.

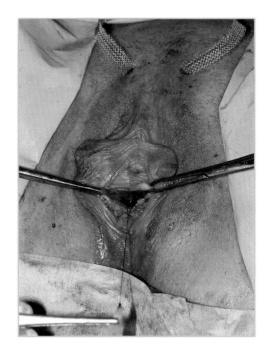

24.15 Thread used for counter-traction.

AFTER OF THE OPERATION

The post-operational stages are:
- procedure with day hospitalisation;
- no urinary catheter;
- no vaginal gauze pad;
- examination of the mictional residue following the first miction: if it is less than 100 cm^3 no further examination is required;
- if the region feels uncomfortable or painful: analgesic drugs for less than 4 days;
- return to sport activity.

OPERATIVE LIFT TECHNIQUE

Just like all other procedures for suburethral slings, the Lift intervention is inspired by and derived from the principle of the suburethral strip as described by Ulmsten and Papapetros. The drive to simplify the procedure resulted in a small number of moderate technical alterations.

Anaesthesia

The anaesthesia will be local or loco-regional, depending on the patient's history, the associated procedures, and the patient's desire. Local anaesthesia is discussed in more detail in the paragraph "Infiltration". Briefly, one uses 1% adrenaline-containing Xylocaïne diluted 1:3 in physiological serum (3 vials containing 20 cm3 each of adrenaline-containing Xylocaïne plus 120 ml physiological serum).

Positioning of the patient, cutaneous asepsis

The patient is installed in a gynaecological position on an operating table that is adapted for operations via a vaginal approach. Her thighs are flexed over abdomen, according to the usual position adapted for vaginal interventions. Usually, gynaecological Betadine will be applied from the knees to the umbilicus. After having carefully washed the vagina, the patient is repositioned, with her legs dipping 15 to 20° below the operating table. Excessive bending of the thighs is not necessary and even dangerous, since it restricts the space where the needles will exit above the pubis and brings the large blood vessels and inguinal fold closer. The operational fields will now be installed using the usual technique.

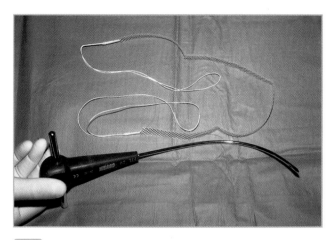

24.16 Material, thread and needle.

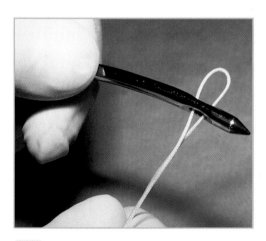

24.17 Thread inserted into the needle's eye.

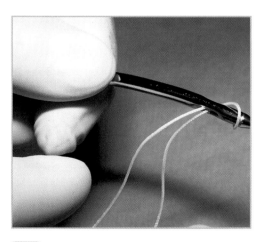

24.18 Thread blocked by a loop around the needle.

Description

Infiltration

A broad infiltration with adrenaline-containing Xylocaïne is advisable so as to facilitate the procedure and prepare the dissection planes, even in the absence of local anaesthesia. This infiltration is realised as follows: 20 cm^3 sub-symphyseally on either side and 20 cm^3 pre-urethrally opposite the incision of the urethra's middle third, all applied via a vaginal approach; 60 cm^3 applied via an abdominal approach retrosymphyseally on either side into the Retzius space. In the rare cases where there is a counter-indication for adrenaline, Xylocaïne or even physiological serum will be used alone with the major goal of preparing the needles' passage and pushing back the bladder by infiltrating the Retzius space. The infiltration points above the pubis are identified with great care, since they will later serve as orientation points during positioning of the needles. Furthermore, if the procedure is performed under local anaesthesia, it is best if the skin and epidermis around the needle's exit point are correctly anaesthetised so as not to cause sharp pain during the needle's cutaneous exit. This point lies strictly above the pubis and about 1 cm on either side of the midline. One must keep in mind that, during the needle's exit, its point comes towards the surgeon, and that the cutaneous exit point often lies strictly opposite the pubic symphysis.

Preparation of the device

While waiting for the local anaesthesia to take effect, the material is prepared (figure 24.16), passing one of the threads attached to the strip's end through the needle's eye (*figure 24.17*). The thread's loop is brought over the needle's point and pulled tight in order to block the thread in place (*figure 24.18*).

Emptying of the Bladder

Before beginning the procedure, the bladder is completely emptied. It does not seem necessary to attempt specific positioning of the bladder during the needles' passage; the infiltration of the space of Retzius is the best insurance against the risk of transvesical puncture.

Incision

One performs an incision of about 1 cm length opposite the urethra's middle third, which is identified and exposed by two Kocher forceps that pull along the vaginal path. This is a firm incision, cutting the vaginal wall in a single gest; the urethra having been pushed back by the infiltration.

Urethro-vaginal dissection

The incision's edges are gripped with an Allis' forceps on either side and the Kocher forceps, which are useless at this stage, are removed. Traction is applied to the forceps in order to create an entry space for the small dissection scissors. The scissors are oriented towards the pubic symphysis and pushed as far as the sub-symphyseal space, verifying with a finger that the vaginal pouch is not perforated. It is not necessary to dissect any further, and the scissors are now opened about 1 cm wide, all the while keeping them within the sub-symphyseal space. The opened scissors are pulled outwards, which enlarges the original dissection path and prepares the needles' passage.

Passage of the needle from both sides

One can now position the *Lift* needles. Traction is again applied to the Allis' forceps and the needle is inserted, on the side one has chosen to commence with, as far as the previously dissected sub-symphyseal space. During this positioning procedure, the needle is oriented along the previously dissected path and positioned laterally without effort. The Allis' forceps are now released and, gripping the needle's base, the needle's point is reoriented towards the midline, targeting the infiltration point located above the pubis about 1-cm from the midline. The skin can be breached without a scalpel incision and the needle is left in place. The same procedure is performed contralaterally.

Cystoscopy

A cystoscopic exam is performed once the thread has been inserted at both sides and before passing the strip through the tissue. If a thread is present inside the bladder, it will have to be removed and repositioned with the help of a needle after having emptied the bladder.

Placing the strip

After having assured the threads' correct position, traction can be applied to the threads (figure 24.20) in order to bring the prosthesis into place suburethrally. One must avoid putting the strip already under tension and must maintain a space of about 1 cm between the urethra and the strip (figure 24.21).

Adjusting the tension during coughing

The strip's tension is adjusted after having filled the bladder with 250 ml physiologic serum. An experienced surgeon can regulate the tension under general anaesthesia without a coughing test. However, in most cases this procedure allows for good efficiency without applying excessive tension. As for the Ulmsten technique, one should ideally allow for a slight urinary leakage and, above all, avoid over adjusting.

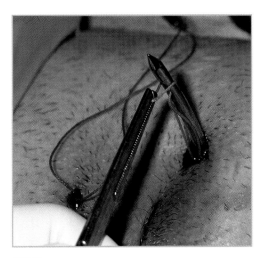

24.20 The thread has been freed and retrieved with a forceps.

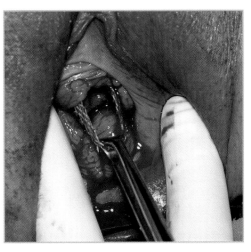

24.21 Counter-traction on the sub-urethral strip.

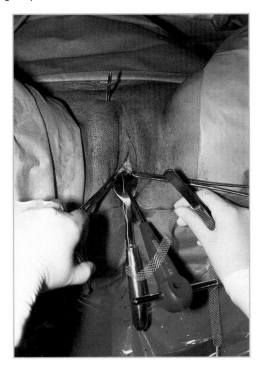

24.19 Needle in place.

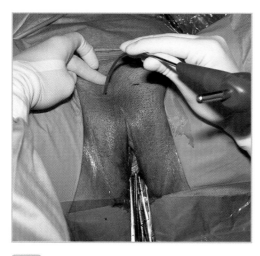

24.22 Passage of the needle from top to bottom on the right.

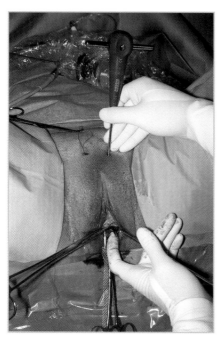

24.23 Needle having exited laterally left of the urethra.

Section of the strip

Once the adjustment has been performed, the strip is sectioned above the pubis at skin level so that the bandage can retract from the cutaneous plane. After having carried out this section, traction is applied with forceps to free the skin's deeper layers, thus assuring good retraction.

Vaginal closure by crossed overcast stitches

The vagina is closed using a no. 1 resorbable thread.

Closure of cutaneous counter-incisions

Finally, the cutaneous plane will be closed with a single stitch of high-resorption thread at the position of each of the cutaneous counter-incisions.

Control of haemostasis

Haemostasis is verified after adjusting the strip. Persistent bleeding might require the putting into place of a vaginal gauze pad and catheter for 24 hours.

Variations in direction of placement

The proposed material's simplicity allows different positioning modes without changing material nor needle. Thus, the needle can be put into place from top to bottom (*figure 24.22 to 24.24*).

One can equally place the strip by a transobturator approach, using a needle with a stronger curvature that is more adapted to the transobturator passage (cf. chapter 25).

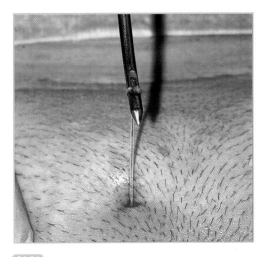

24.24 Retrieving the thread through the cutaneous incision.

Suburethral slings via a transobturator approach

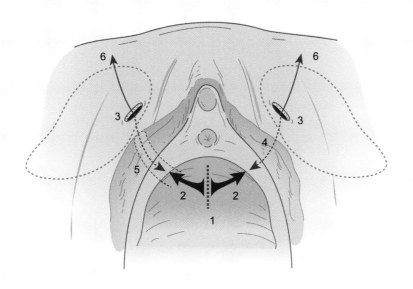

25.1 *Summary sketch.*
1. Vaginal incision. 2. Lateral dissection towards the obturator orifice. 3. Cutaneous incision opposite the obturator orifice. 4. Passage of the needles. 5. Positioning the prosthesis. 6. Adjusting the tension.

Guide to the reader

1. Recall the anatomy of the obturator orifice and of the vascular and nervous pedicles, as well as of the viscera that are in close contact.
2. List the individual operational stages for placement of the subureteral slings via a transobturator approach.
3. Name the different techniques including cystocele treatment using a prosthesis using the same access route.

The transobturator suspension is based on the passage of a needle originating from the obturator orifice and through the pelvic aponeurosis. The suspension relies on the blocking of the prosthesis in the median pelvic aponeurosis, which is often thin and of variable stability on its own, but sufficiently strong if a wide prosthesis is put into place. Since Delorme described its use in the treatment of incontinence, its application has spread widely. The theoretical benefit of using this access route for placing a sub-ureteral prosthesis is the highly reduced risk of incurring vesical injury. Furthermore, this access route is relatively harmless, since the vascular and nervous pedicles are distant.

DESCRIPTION

The technique described here is a treatment for urinary incontinence by placing a subureteral prosthesis via the trans-obturator access route.

Similarities to other techniques for urinary incontinence treatment using a subureteral sling are numerous. We will not describe the preparatory stages again in detail, but instead indicate the relevant chapters. This concerns the vaginal incision, as well as the vaginal dissection, which will be more extensive than usual in order to allow the passage of an index finger through the paravesical fossae to reach the obturator orifice. This modification is, it should be noted, prejudicial to both the reproducibility and the quality of the result, since it requires a more extensive incision and subureteral dissection. This dissection can be responsible for a secondary mobility of the vaginal strip's subureteral portion, particularly in the direction of the uterovesical junction.

Infiltration, vaginal incision and vaginal dissection

The incision is identified by two Kocher forceps and the incision is preceded by a local infiltration. As indicated above, the incision is about 2 cm long across from the middle third of the urethra, but extended towards the uretro-vesical junction, without quite reaching this latter junction. Similarly, the dissection, begun using scissors, is directed towards the paravesical spaces and is enlarged enough in order to allow the surgeon's finger to enter. By inserting a finger onto the paravesical fossa,

one can palpate the obturator orifice and lead the needle with a finger to prevent injury to the bladder.

Cutaneous incision opposite the obturator orifice

The obturator orifice is wide and its lower part, at a safe distance from the vasculo-nervous obturator pedicle, can be passed through from its inside portion. The original description of the obturator incision recommended the use of an orientation point located 2 cm laterally and 1 cm below the urethra. Such an access is indeed easy, but does not appear optimal for the treatment of urinary incontinence because of the low-positioned urethral support it provides. On several occasions, we were faced with patients whose urinary incontinence was not corrected, even after the prosthesis was put under maximal tension. Worse still, persistent post-operative incontinence required a second procedure, applying the classical technique through the Retzius space...

Following Bernard Jacquetin's and Georges Mellier's suggestions, we therefore prefer to only use this location for the placement of subvesical prostheses in the case of cystocele treatment. Urinary incontinence is better treated using an incision that is placed further up, lateral to the clitoris, in order to obtain improved support (*figure 25.2*). This incision should be about 3 mm long in order to allow passage of the needle.

Passage of the needle led by the finger

The needle must be adapted to the anatomy of the obturator orifice and, therefore, possess a large, hooked curvature in order to allow this passage without having to have the handle jammed against the thigh (*figure 25.3*).

As soon as the deeper plane is breached, the needle can be felt through the obturator orifice. At this first stage, it is

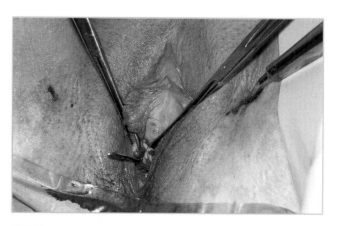

25.2 Cutaneous incision across from the obturator orifice.

important to get past the bony branch by penetrating 1 to 2 cm before passing alongside this branch white turning around it in the direction of the obturator orifice. The needle's point is palpated by the surgeon's index finger, which then accompanies its rotation. The point is thus led all the way to the vaginal incision. This action must be further extended in order to expose the needle's eye. Passing the prosthesis or its traction thread through the needle's eye is thus facilitated.

Attention: one must avoid pushing the needle too far when bypassing the pubic branch during passage through the obturator orifice; there is a risk of injury to the obturator pedicle, and, above all, a risk of injury to the bladder. The latter might entail the necessity of performing cytoscopic examination while training for the technique.

One must make sure that the needle does not pass through the lateral vaginal pouch and that the needle's point does not come into close contact with the urethra, which could cause injury to it.

Placing the thread or prosthesis in the needle

The prosthesis' arm, or a thread attached to it, is slid into the needle's eye. The needle can now be pulled back and both ends of the prosthesis recovered (*figure 25.4*).

Adjusting the tension

The tension can be adjusted without difficulties and should ideally be performed in a conscious patient. The bladder should be filled with 250 cm^3 (*figure 25.5*) as described for other suburethral slings (*chapter 24*).

Section of the prosthesis, closure of the incisions

After having adjusted the tension, the prosthesis is stretched to skin level and sectioned at the surface of the skin. The incision will be closed with a resorbable stitch. The vaginal incision in closed with an overcast suture.

NORMAL SURGICAL REPERCUSSIONS

In the absence of complications, the procedure can be performed based on a single day of hospitalisation. Following the first miction, it is desirable to examine the mictional residue.

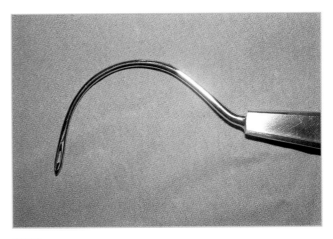

25.3 Passage of the needle under finger control. Needle with a large curvature for a transobturator passage.

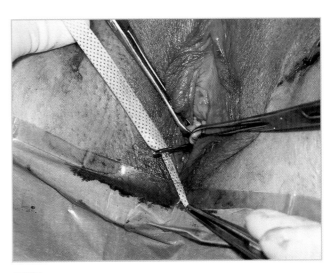

25.4 Placing the prosthesis in the needle.

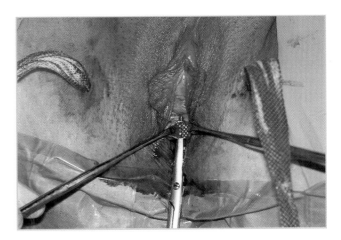

25.5 Adjusting the tension.

CHAPTER 26

Vaginal sling

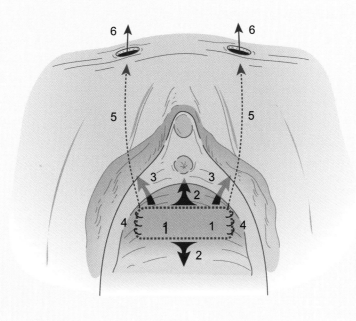

26.1 *Summary sketch.*
1. Incision of the vaginal strip. 2. Dissection of the incision's edges in anticipation of the closure. 3. Lateral dissection. 4. The sutures laterally grasp the vaginal strip. 5. Passing the threads through the Retzius space. 6. Adjusting the tension.

Guide to the reader

1. Discuss the indications for vaginal strips.
2. List the technical details that differentiate it from the Bologna operation.

The "vaginal sling" has been described by Gilles Crépin. It refers to a transversal vaginal strip of about 2 cm height and 5 to 6 cm length, prepared at the uretro-vesical junction. Although this procedure is extremely simple to perform and of negligible cost, it presents several major disadvantages. Not least of which is the risk of a secondary mucocele linked to the enclosing of vaginal tissue – as also seen in the case of a plastron – which is why this procedure should be reserved for menopausal patients. Furthermore, the results in case of treatment for isolated urinary incontinence have not yet been sufficiently evaluated. We, therefore, only apply this procedure to menopausal patients that present a urinary incontinence under stress together with an associated prolapse. In contrast to the Bologna intervention, this technique does not require that the patient present an associated cystocele (resection of vaginal tissue is very limited). Today, one must also apply the procedures used during the placement of suburethral slings, i.e. adjustment of the strip's tension under loco-regional anaesthesia in order to diminish the risk of urinary retention and of a secondary dysuria. The vaginal strip can easily be prepared to the detriment of the vagina, positioned across from the middle third of the urethra, as described previously for these slings.

DESCRIPTION

Position identification of the vaginal strip and placement of the Kocher forceps

At a first stage, the vaginal strip's position, which should be about 2 cm high and 3 cm wide, is identified. The Kocher forceps delimit the vaginal incision.

Vaginal infiltration

The infiltration is performed in relation to the incision, but not below the vaginal strip, which remains adherent, and then laterally along the dissection's path towards the Retzius space.

This infiltration must enable a dissection that is sufficient to allow a finger to pass. It can be extended to the Retzius space.

Vesical incision and dissection

Following a firm incision of the vagina, the Allis' forceps are positioned, two on the upper and two on the lower edges of the incision. Traction exerted on the Allis' forceps allows the presentation of the dissection spaces in order to liberate about 1 cm below the upper edge and 1–2 cm on the lower edge (figure 26.2).

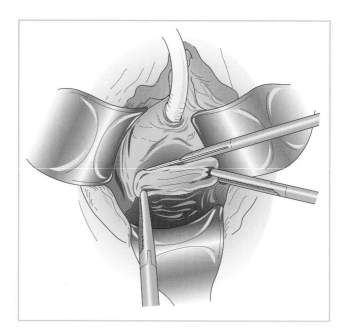

26.2 Incision of the vaginal strip.

Vesicovaginal dissection

The dissection is now extended laterally to the bladder's sides, towards the branches of the pubic symphysis. It is not necessary to extend this dissection any further than required to allow passage of the surgeon's finger.

Accessing the Retzius space

Having reached the branches of the pubic symphysis, one proceeds with the opening of the paravesical fossae by perforating them with scissors. The vaginal strip is taken hold of with two non-resorbable threads (figure 26.3) (cf. chapter 27, "Intervention of Bologna".)

Passage of the non-resorbable threads through the Retzius space

The threads are grasped with a Bengolea forceps, which, lying alongside the surgeon's finger in order to protect the bladder, is brought into contact with the abdominal aponeurosis. A cutaneous incision, as well as an incision of the aponeurosis are performed across from the position of each of the forceps, and the threads are brought to the surface of the skin. The threads of the vaginal strip's two ends are brought together along the midline and tied while regulating the tension as described for the synthetic sub-urethral slings (figure 26.4).

Regulating the sling's tension and vaginal closure

After having regulated the sling's tension, one proceeds with the vaginal closure. The intervention is terminated by verification of haemostasis and a count of compresses.

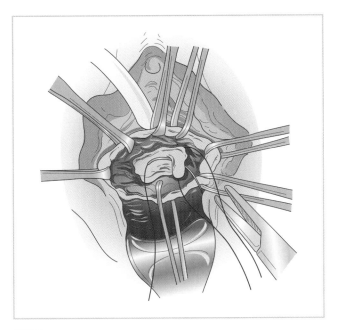

26.3 Vaginal strip taken hold of with the needle.

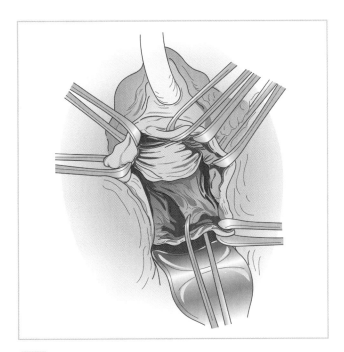

26.4 Suspension threads passed through the Retzius space.

CHAPTER 27

Bologna operation

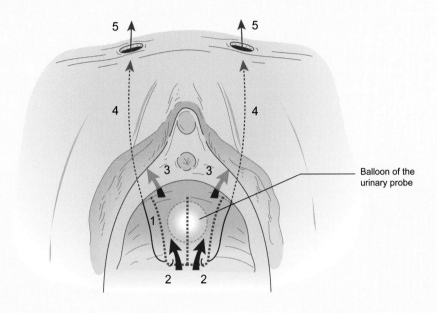

Balloon of the
urinary probe

27.1 *Summary sketch.*
1. Incision of the vaginal strips. 2. Dissection of the strips. 3. Vesical dissection. 4. Passage of the threads through the Retzius space. 5. Adjusting the tension.

Guide to the reader

1. Name the main operation stages.
2. Distinguish the operational stages for incontinence treatment from those for cystocele treatment.
3. Detail the techniques for accessing and crossing of the space of Retzius.
4. Identify the differences between this intervention and the positioning of a "classical" sling.

The Bologna operation consists of producing a sling of vaginal tissue from excessive anterior vaginal tissue related to the presence of an associated cystocele. This sling is inserted at the level of the urethro-vesical junction and consists of two vaginal strips that are about 2 cm wide and 5 to 7 cm long. These strips, which have their foothold across from the urethro-vesical junction, are suspended to the abdominal aponeurosis by a short suprapubic counter-incision with use of a non-resorbable suture. At the moment, the general consensus is that the strip must not be brought above the abdominal aponeurosis during suspension, due to a few reports cases of mucocele. For this same reason, we prefer to perform this intervention in menopausal patients—as is the case with all techniques that involve enclosing of vaginal tissue—due to the subsequent risk of mucocele.

INDICATIONS

The Bologna intervention is indicated:
– if urinary incontinence during stress has been confirmed;
– if the urinary incontinence is debilitating or is masked by the cystocele;
– if urinary incontinence is associated with a cystocele with excess anterior vaginal tissue;
– for menopausal patients.

RELATED INTERVENTIONS

Classical slings of the urethro-vesical junction as well as the vaginal sling have several operational stages in common with the Bologna intervention, especially those concerning the passage through the Retzius space and adjusting the tension.

DESCRIPTION

The procedure described here is the treatment of stress incontinence in association with a cystocele.

Positioning the Kocher forceps

While positioning the Kocher forceps, one must anticipate the shape and size of the vaginal strips. The median incision is simple to prepare, but the strips' width has direct consequences for the vaginal resection, for possible difficulties during secondary vaginal closure and for a possible narrowing of the vagina. Therefore, this preparatory operational stage must not be skipped; it provides the possibility to trace a imaginary incision, the consequences of which will be directly assessed. Thus, the Kocher forceps are positioned across from the strips' lateral protrusion on the upper part, located at the level of the urethro-vesical junction, and on the lower part, located at the level of the pericervical incision in the case of an associated hysterectomy. The position of the urethro-vesical junction is estimated by palpation of the bulge of the vesical probe that is pulled downwards. The lateral forceps are brought towards each other on the midline in order to evaluate the tension that will exist following the final vaginal closure.

Vaginal infiltration and incision

Here, the vaginal infiltration is performed into the depth of the vaginal tissue, below the future vaginal strips, in order to facilitate the dissection in the deeper planes, and laterally towards the pubic branches, in order to allow vesical dissection and to prepare the access to the Retzius space. One could equally infiltrate the Retzius space, but its dissection from top to bottom using a finger largely reduces the risk of a vesical wound. We, therefore, do not find that a systemic infiltration of the Retzius space to be necessary.

The incision will be pericervical and "T"-shaped in the case of an associated hysterectomy. In the anterior vaginal wall this incision runs medially at first, starting at the urethro-vesical junction – identified as indicated previously – as far as the limit of the pericervical incision or the vaginal floor. One imme-

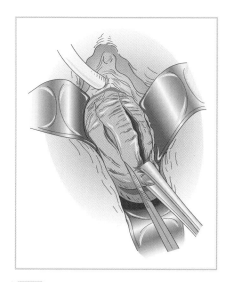

27.2 Incision of the vaginal strips.

diately performs the incision of the two vaginal strips (*figure 27.2*), although their dissection can be postponed until after a possible hysterectomy.

Vesicovaginal dissection

This dissection stage can be postponed until after the vaginal hysterectomy, in order to diminish the nuisance that a slow, persistent bleeding might represent. The dissection begins with that of the two strips, grasping a strip's free end and following the dissection plane with the bladder with a cold scalpel, facilitated by the preceding infiltration (*figure 27.3*). The dissection is extended laterally by putting under traction the Allis' forceps that are holding the edges of the lateral incision. It is initiated with a cold scalpel and continued with a finger padded by a compress. This operational stage is identical to that described during Campbell's intervention (*cf.* chapter 14).

Retropubic dissection and access to the Retzius space

The Retzius space is accessed via the lower side of the pubic branches. The paravesical fossae, having been opened, are not enlarged laterally as is done when one wishes to dissect the tendinous arches of the pelvic fascia. Here it is absolutely sufficient to continue the dissection with a finger, breaching the middle pelvic aponeurosis in the direction of the Retzius space.

Passage of the vaginal strips through the Retzius space

Before passing the vaginal strips through the Retzius space, a non-resorbable, transfixing thread is passed through each of the strips, confirming a sufficient length, while leaving the strip's free end just below the plane of the abdominal aponeurosis (*figure 27.4*). As discussed for classical slings, the thread can be either passed from top to bottom or from bottom to top; however, the needle or thread-carrying forceps must be guided by the surgeon's right index finger (if he is right-handed) in order to protect the bladder. The two threads are recovered by the same, about 2-cm-long, median counter-incision performed at the level of the midline. The thread having been put under traction, the strip can easily by made to rise inside the Retzius space (*figure 27.5*). In case of doubt concerning an possible urinary problems, a cystoscopy, with or without injection of blue dye, is advisable in order to adapt the following stages accordingly and repeat the passage of the strips, should the bladder have been perforated.

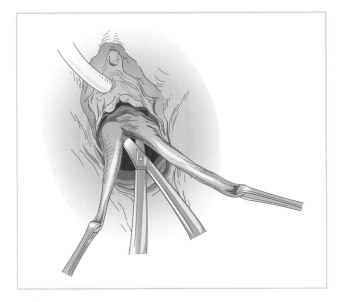

27.3 Dissection of the vaginal strips.

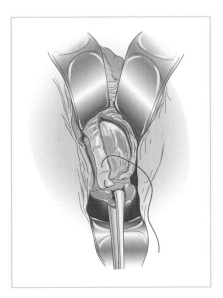

27.4 Non-resorbable thread carried by a needle is passed through the vaginal strip.

In the case of a bladder wound
One verifies by cystoscopy.

A bladder suture is usually not possible, since the wound occurs on the bladder's ventral side, outside the reach of the vaginal route.

First of all, the bladder must be emptied and the once again the threads passed through the Retzius space, this time making sure that the passage does not transfix the bladder. Since the dissection is more important than during placement of a synthetic suburethral sling, a urinary catheter with free drainage is put into place during a period of three to four days.

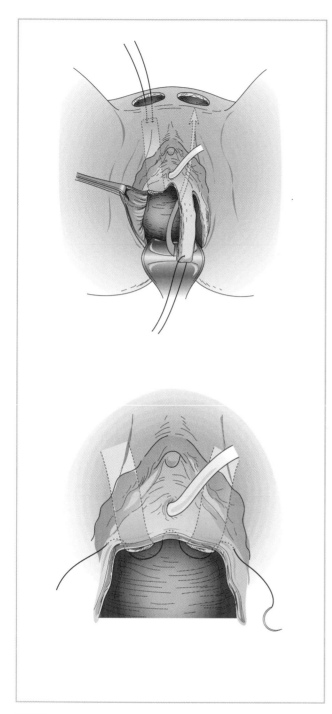

27.5 Passage of the vaginal strips through the Retzius space.

Cystocele treatment, with or without association with vaginal hysterectomy

In most instances in which a hysterectomy is associated, treatment of an associated cystocele consists of a sub-symphyseal crossing of the uterosacral ligaments according to Campbell's procedure. A paravaginal suspension can only be associated if the remaining vaginal surface is sufficient to allow closure without tension of the anterior colporraphy.

Closing the anterior colporraphy

The vaginal closure is achieved with a crossed overcast suture after having verified haemostasis and counted the compresses.

Haemorrhage

In the case of persistent haemorrhage originating from inside the Retzius space, a thick vaginal gauze is put into place for 24 hours, a urinary catheter with free drainage is left in place, clamped postoperatively for two hours, after having injected 200 cm^3 into the bladder.

Adjusting the tension of the vaginal strips' suspension

The vaginal strips' tension is adjusted at the end of the procedure, ideally in a manner similar to other sling techniques, i.e., under loco-regional anaesthesia. The two non-resorbable threads, recovered via a short median counter-incision of 2 cm length above the pubis, are knotted together above the abdominal aponeurosis. Having filled the bladder with 200 cm^3 physiologic serum, the patient is made to cough and the tension is increased until the urinary leakages are corrected. Here, it is not indispensable to consider a minimal urinary leakage, since the autologous tissue can be distended secondarily more easily if necessary. However, this precaution allows one to diminish the risk of a postoperative retention, or even dysuria. The counter-incision is subsequently closed with an intradermic suture using a highly resorbable thread (*figure 27.5*).

CHAPTER 28

"Classical" slings

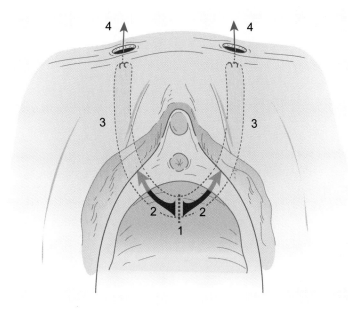

28.1 *Summary sketch.*
1. Incision 1-cm opposite the middle third of the urethra. 2. Lateral dissection. 3. Passage of the needles.
4. Adjusting the tension.

Guide to the reader

1. Describe the different variations of existing slings and their general principles.
2. List the respective advantages and disadvantages of these procedures.
3. Detail the different operational stages, particularly the passage technique through the Retzius space.

*B*ased on the principle of directly suspending the uterovesical junction, the efficiency of these techniques is in part due to the obstructive effect resulting from the tension applied. This obstructive effect is the reason for preferring the use of such techniques e.g. in the case of a sphincter insufficiency. However, the same effect is also the cause of a prolonged urinary retention, as well as of debilitating secondary dysuria. The slings that are nowadays referred to as "classical slings", together with the colposuspensions according to Burch, represent the main reference techniques for treatment of urinary incontinence occurring under stress…in the pre-"TVT" world. Since then, the new religion has, in the view of many surgeons, turned these procedures into peripheral surgical techniques. Without doubt, the progressive evaluation of secondary complications associated with suburethral slings, as well as of their failures, will do justice to these earlier techniques that are easy to perform while providing favourable long-term results. However, some technical modifications and complementary evaluations might have to be performed.

The results published for theses techniques are comparable to those achieved with colposuspension techniques, and it is merely the absence of randomised studies that has prevented them from obtaining their precise place among urinary incontinence treatments.

VARIATIONS

Numerous techniques for different types of slings have been described, varying in the material used (synthetic or autologous), the technique for adjusting the tension, and in the access route used in order to put the sling into place.

We will not describe the classical Goebell-Stoeckel operations with application of a musculo-aponeurotic strip: we do not have any experience with this technique and their postoperative morbidity has progressively reduced the scope of their indications, even though they produce encouraging results concerning urinary continence.

Variations in the use of materials

Variations are found in the material used for the sling itself, which can be autologous, removed from the aponeurosis or from the patient's thigh (fascia lata), or originating from the cadaver (fascia lata, dura mater), with all the legitimate

reservations this requires in terms of virological security. One can use vaginal tissue, as described in chapter 26 "Vaginal slings", with reservations concerning long-term efficiency for the treatment of isolated incontinence.

Variations in the passage through the Retzius space

Most of the sling techniques commence with a vaginal incision that is directly followed by a dissection and breaching of the Retzius space via the vaginal route using a finger. Some surgeons prefer to then glide a forceps via the vaginal access along their finger, protecting the bladder. Others will rather perforate the abdominal aponeurosis with a needle, such as a Stamey needle, directly on the surgeon's finger, which will then guide it all the way to the vaginal incision. These do not represent individual techniques, but rather personal preferences.

We lastly consider the techniques for regulating the slings's tension, a major part of the procedure. Ideally, this adjustment should be performed under loco-regional anaesthesia. It should be adapted to the correct exactly of any urinary leakage of the coughing patient with the bladder filled. Blind adjustment of the tension must be avoided, leading to the risk of over-adjusteing that could result in prolonged urinary retention. If adjustment is performed under general anaesthesia, one must resist the temptation of "good intentions" and not apply tension. Ideally, the knot will be left free, so that it can be lifted 1 to 2 cm above the aponeurosis after having been pulled tight.

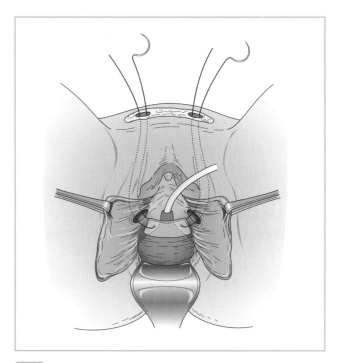

28.2 Vaginal sling procedure using sub-cervical strips suspended to the anterior abdominal wall by a mixed approach.

INDICATIONS

The classical slings are indicated for:
– a urinary incontinence during stress;
– one that has been confirmed by examination, with a pad-test and during the urodynamic evaluation;
– debilitating urinary incontinences or those hidden by a cystocele;
– patients of all ages.

DESCRIPTION

The technique described here is a treatment for isolated urinary incontinence (figure 28.2).

Identifying the urethro-vesical junction and positioning the Kocher forceps

The urethro-vesical junction is identified by the bulge of the vesical probe that has been filled and pulled downward, so that it can serve to identify the junction by palpation. Ideally, the functional, as opposed to the anatomical, junction has previously been identified by vaginal ultrasound including an exact measurement of the distance from the junction to the urethral orifice. The Kocher forceps mark off the vaginal incision and are positioned on either side of the vaginal incision, transversally about 5 cm from each other.

Vaginal infiltration

The infiltration is performed below the incision and laterally along the dissection path towards the Retzius space. This infiltration must allow for a dissection that is sufficient to allow passage of a finger. The infiltration can be extended into the Retzius space.

Incision and dissection of the junction

The vaginal incision is followed by positioning the Allis' forceps, two on the upper edge and two on the lower edge. Traction exerted on the Allis' forceps displays the dissection spaces, allowing the liberation of 1 cm below the upper edge and 1 to 2 cm above the lower edge.

Vesicovaginal dissection

The dissection is now extended laterally to the bladder's sides, towards the branches of the pubic symphysis. It is unnecessary to dissect more than required to allow passage of the surgeon's finger.

Access to the Retzius space

Having reached the point opposite to the branches of the pubic symphysis, one proceeds by opening the paravesical fossae, perforating them with scissors (cf. chapter 27, Bologna). The strip is taken hold of with two non-resorbable threads.

Passage of the non-resorbable threads through the Retzius space

The threads are gripped with a Bengolea forceps, which is brought into contact with the abdominal aponeurosis, all the while moving along the surgeon's finger, thus protecting the bladder. A cutaneous incision as well as an incision of the aponeurosis is carried out opposite each of the forceps, and the threads are brought to the skin. The threads coming from the vaginal strips are brought together at the midline and tied, adjusting the tension as previously described for the sub-urethral strips.

Putting the strip into place and attaching opposite the junction

In order to avoid a secondary mobilisation of the strip below the urethra, one can easily fix the strip to the para-urethral tissues with two stitches using resorbable thread.

Adjusting the strip tension and vaginal closure

The tension is adjusted as described in the chapter that is devoted to the Bologna intervention (cf. chapter 27). One then proceeds with the vaginal closure.

The intervention is completed with a verification of haemostasis and a count of compresses.

Diagnosis and treatment of complications

PART 7

CHAPTER 29

Visceral injury

Guide to the reader

1. As for all complications, methods for both prevention and taking care of visceral injury must be considered.
2. Prevention forms the basis of all expository and preparatory procedures. Its goal is not only to provide the surgeon with a large field of view, but also to allow him to work with the anatomy in order to distance the organs at risk.
3. If visceral lesions are immediately taken care of, a complication can be turned into a mere incident. The great majority of visceral injuries can be handled by the same surgeon and during the same operational session. Should the gynaecological surgeon not feel sufficiently competent, he should not hesitate to ask for advice from a urological or visceral surgeon.

BLADDER INJURY

The bladder is at risk during vaginal surgery, with a significant rate of vesical injury, which is fortunately without consequence if identified and treated immediatly. If ignored, however, they can be the source of postoperative fistulas.

During simple vaginal hysterectomy, protection of the bladder is exclusively achieved by the anatomical identification of the "supravaginal wall" (cf. chapter 4), which is firmly sectioned just after its unambiguous identification. Causes of bladder injury are:

– scissors taking a errant path when breaching the supravaginal wall: remember to section halfway between the edge of the vagina and the uterine isthmus;

– penetration with the finger, which is not advisable as long as the vesicouterine septum has not been reached;

– specific adhesions resulting from a previous surgical intervention.

During radical hysterectomy or colpectomy, the difficulties are more acute, as the vesical recess is more marked and the supravaginal wall appears thicker, since it is enhanced with fibres terminating at the vagina. During cystocele surgery, the recess is large by definition, while the vesical wall is extremely thin and the vaginal wall often impaired, even without considering the fact that surgical interventions can be frequent. In such cases, we advise a primary complete dissection of the cystocele pocket on the midline, the vesicouterine septum and the peritoneal pouch.

Prevention, other than anatomical precautions, can be improved by placing a Béniqué probe if particular difficulties are encountered. An indwelling catheter is not advised: it is better to slightly fill the bladder so that the dissection plane becomes more visible, and allowing bladder injury to be identified by a characteristic leaking. Leaking will be even more visible if a coloured liquid (usually methylene blue) is injected into the bladder at the beginning of the intervention.

Lesions of the blader do not qualify as a major accident. We choose to repair such injury following the exeresis stage: good access to the bladder helps to avoid further injury. Any doubt or particular difficulty must be checked with a blue-dye test at the end of the procedure, but before vaginal closure. A gauze pad is placed inside the peritoneum and about 300 ml coloured liquid are instilled into the bladder. The gauze pad is removed and the absence of dye is verified.

Repair is usually easy. A couple of rules is necessary and sufficient:

– the total-plane approach using a slowly resorbable thread is the most reliable method, an extramucous suture representing a probably useless sophistication;

– this plane must be perfectly water-tight, this being verified with a dye test;

– every leak must be blocked shut, a second plane being required only if water-tightness is not achieved;

– vesical drainage of large calibre (20 French units) is required over a period of time that varies according to the size of the injury (three days for a simple puncture, five to seven days for a larger wound).

If the lesion is not median and close to the orifices and intramural paths of the ureters, repair may be difficult. The ureters can be palpated inside the detrusor, following the palpation procedure described for Schauta operation. If necessary, the orifices can be identified and catheterised. It is imperative that the stitches applied avoid any risk of stenosis or significant bending of the intramural ureters.

INJURY TO THE URETHRA

Urethral injury is rare and complicates treatment of prolapse or urinary incontinence. It can be repaired during the operation, either via vaginal or abdominal access, using a supporting probe. Unidentified injuries lead to uretrovaginal fistula. A highly positioned intrasphincter fistula results in permanent incontinence and requires difficult surgical treatment with interposition of a cutaneous, fatty, or vesical flap. A low-positioned sub-sphincter fistula only results in post-mictional incontinence and is easily treated by excision and suture with use of a probe.

INJURY TO THE URETER

During vaginal surgery, a ureteral wound is rare, but possible. As during abdominal surgery, the ureter is at risk:

– during haemostasis of the uterine artery;

– during haemostasis of the ovarian pedicle;

– during difficult dissections of the broad ligament or if a tumour is enclosed inside the broad ligament;

– while preparing the ureter during radical hysterectomy.

Furthermore, there is a risk during treatment of all externalised prolapses specific to vaginal surgery: sectioning during dissection of the cystocele. Finally, difficulties are also encountered due to congenital anomalies: ureterocele and, above all, a bifid or duplicated ureter, not always identified preoperatively, since urography is not a standard preoperative procedure for gynaecological operations.

Prevention

Many basic actions of surgeons are performed with the aim to prevent ureteral traumatisms, and all of them are important. They are based on two anatomical principles: the retroligamental ureter is positioned against the pelvic wall, while the sub- and preligamental ureter is located inside the "bladder pillar".

The *retroligamentous* ureter, at risk during haemostasis of the ovarian pedicles, is protected from the clamping of the pedicle via a vaginal approach if, and only if, the adnexa can be distanced from the pelvic wall. One must, therefore, try by all means to create pediculed adnexa by pulling towards the midline: the ureter is never pulled along by this action, thus providing space for a clamp (*figure 29.1*). If this is impossible to perform, one will have to chose another access route. This is the case with ovaries that are high up, or retracted against the wall due to an infectious pathology, as a result of previous surgery, or due to age. The same is true in cases of adnexial pathologies with adhesions (endometriosis, sequels to infection or surgery), which fix the ovaries to the posterior side of the broad ligament. If the adhesions can be detached via a vaginal approach, the normal anatomical situation can be reconstituted. Should this not be the case, vaginal adnexectomy will not be possible.

If an accidental avulsion of the ovary should occur, haemostasis can only be performed if the pedicle can be grasped with a dissection forceps to provide space for a clamp or a Roeder loop (Endoloop, cf. figure 30.4). If this is not possible, haemostasis must be performed by laparoscopy or laparotomy. Under no circumstances should toothed clamps be used to check the ovarian pedicle, nor coagulations, nor blind "X" stitches nor a blind hold. A diagnosis carried out during the operation concerning ureter traumatism in this anatomical situation is practically impossible and must be repaired via a laparotomy.

The *subligamentous* ureter can be injured during the course of a simple hysterectomy, prolapse surgery and radical hysterectomy.

Haemostasis of the uterine artery during total simple hysterectomy must be established within the bladder pillar. This ensures that it is also established within the ureter, which itself forms part of the bladder pillar. The pillar must, therefore, be pushed away laterally with the help of two retractors: at this stage, the assistant surgeon is more important than the surgeon, and the latter's role is to help the assistant surgeon in correctly placing the retractors. The retractor must be inserted into the vesicouterine space and pushed laterally and imperturbably towards the side where the uterine artery is being treated (*figures 29.2 to 29.4*); in an ideal setting, the uterine artery will be visible, so that the surgeon does not have to grip blindly. To do this, the vesicouterine septum must have been opened correctly, in the adequate plane displaying the uterine fascia and, if possible, the anterior peritoneal pouch at the far end of the detachment.

A tumour of the broad ligament represents a special case, since it can result in the ureter's artificial displacement to a level below that of the uterine artery. A fixed or malignant tumour is an indication for laparotomy. A large, non-fixed tumour can be treated by laparoscopic preparation, while a small, non-fixed tumour can be removed via a vaginal approach. In both cases, the procedure must be absolutely restricted to an enucleation of a benign tumour within its cleavage plane. This is the best approach to avoid lesion both to the ureter that has been pushed out of the way and to the peripheral blood vessels, for which random haemostasis could result in a ureteral traumatism.

In prolapse surgery

One must consider the possibility of a ureter prolapse. The above rules have to be applied, especially the correct opening of the vesicouterine septum, but two further precautions have to be followed:

– a laterally extended vesicouterine separation achieved by section of what prolapse surgeons improperly refer to as the "bladder pillar", although it merely represents the pillar's medial part. Since, in contrast to a Watkin's (or Schauta) operation, there is no need to directly observe the ureter, only the uterine insertion of this structure is sectioned by remaining in contact with the uterus;

– the palpation of the ureter inside the downwardly distended pillar; here, the procedures described for prolapse treatment and radical vaginal hysterectomy are combined: the vesicouterine septum is opened, deepened and enlarged (this is the recurring theme for all uterine surgery via a vaginal approach), the anterior colpocele is detached laterally (resulting in opening of the Latzko's paravesical fossae if the manoeuvre is performed in sufficient depth, e.g., as for preparation of a paravaginal suspension during a Watkin's

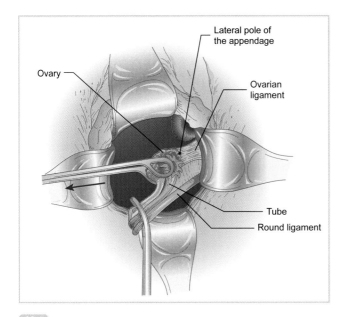

Ovary

Lateral pole of the appendage

Ovarian ligament

Tube

Round ligament

29.1 The ureter is distanced from the appendage by pulling towards the midline.

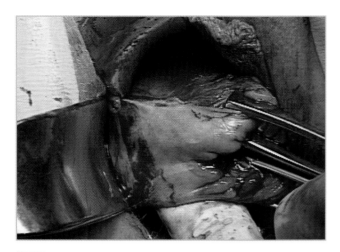

29.2 Prevention of ureteral traumatism by proper arrangement of the anterior retractor.

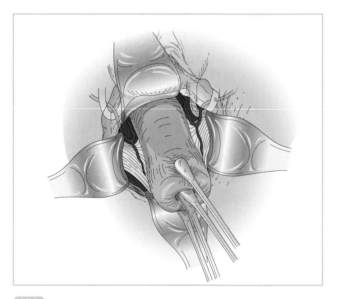

29.3 Placement of the retractor in order to protect the ureter by distancing the "bladder pillar". Surgical view.
Rotation of the retractor towards the patient's right side protects the right ureter by pushing the bladder's pillar away laterally (see also Watkin's technique, chapter 10, in order to better understand this structure); the uterine artery's loop has been displayed. On the patient's left side, the retractor does not protect the ureter, and the uterine artery's loop is closed; in order to treat the left side, the retractor will have to be moved towards the left side, while applying rightward traction to the uterine cervix.

operation); the true bladder pillar is thus defined, a thick structure delimiting the two new spaces.   The ureter can now be palpated inside the pillar, either between two fingers or a finger and a retractor placed on the pillar's opposite side (*figure 29.5*).

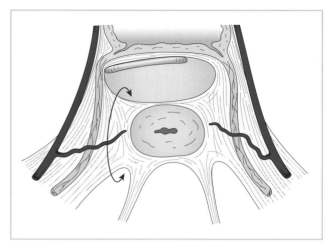

29.4 Placement of the retractor for protecting the ureter by distancing the "bladder pillar". View in section. The arrow designates the passage of the haemostasis thread, which takes hold of the uterus and cardinal ligament (paracervix), within which the ureter that has been properly distanced.

In *Watkin's radical hysterectomy*, identification and distancing of the subligamental ureter are part of the surgical protocol. Taking the wrong passage during this delicate stage can result in lesions to the ureter. The most dangerous scenario is the misinterpretation of a palpated structure as the ureter and, as a result, the sectioning of the true ureter while separating the pillar's contents. The most confusing scenario is encountered if the ureter's lowest point has not been identified: if the ureter's "knee" has been identified correctly, it marks the point below which there will be no ureter; and erroneous interpretation of its position can lead to an accidental sectioning of the ureter. Another delicate stage is at the end of the surgical intervention, during which the uterosacral ligaments are definitively sectioned at their distal position relative to the uterus. Whether this gesture is performed from bottom to top or from top to bottom after a Doderlein manoeuvre, the ureter's retro-ligamental part is under threat of lesion, having been pulled downwards together with the peritoneum to which it adheres.

Treatment

Post-operative diagnosis and treatment of ureteral traumatisms do not lie within the scope of this book. The intraoperative treatment is by far the most desirable: the lesion is fresh and easily identifiable, and the patient has been warned of a urinary risk inherent to all gynaecological operations – as is done systematically.

A simple pinching of the ureter, for a short time and without visible attrition does not require any treatment. A more prolonged, non-penetrating pinching leaving visible lesions justifies the placement of a ureteral probe, either systematically during the operation, or after identification of a renal distension and the failure of corticoid treatment. The intraoperative solution, by placing an endoprosthesis under cystoscopic control, appears preferable and is better tolerated by the patient.

Under favourable anatomical conditions, a lateral ureter wound must be sutured onto a probe via vaginal approach. This is often the case if the view is sufficient to allow diagnosis of a lateral wound. The (simple J) ureteral probe is left inside the bladder and retrieved after cicatrisation, a good 12 days after the intervention (figures 29.6 and 29.7).

Complete section of the ureter can be repaired via a vaginal or abdominal approach. Traditionally, the abdominal approach is used: it is indicated if the technical conditions are not favourable, i.e., if the vaginal access is too narrow, or if the lesion is situated too far up. It is true that during vaginal surgery the majority of ureteral lesions are observed at the level of the subligamental ureter, in a place where the uterovesical reimplantation is considered most secure, but where one can attempt a suture via a vaginal approach in order to avoid a laparotomy. We will merely describe this technique via the vaginal approach (figures 29.5 and 29.6). It should only be considered if the lesion is perfectly visible, providing the conditions for a high quality suture onto a guiding probe. Placing a probe inside the two extremities represents the procedure's first stage. The lower segment must be catheterised as far as the bladder, the upper segment as far as the pelvis using a probe with a sufficient calibre (generally 5 to 7 French units). A tight, extra-mucous suture is then applied using a slow resorption thread. The after-effects include the risk of a fistula and, above all, of a stenosis that might require either endoscopic treatment or conventional surgery. Prevention of such complications is based on insuring good vascularisation of the anastomosed segments (including the absence of coagulation), as well as on strictly atraumatic manipulations in general.

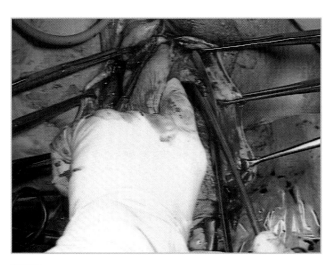

29.5 Neat ureteral section.
In the case of a large prolapse, opening of the spaces must precede any latero-vesical section. This step, using scissors, has resulted in ureteral section. A posteriori, it is evident that the paravesical fossa should have been opened all the way up to the contact point with the forceps at the image's top right, and to detach only that space without sectioning anything – except if the ureter has been palpated in what turns out to be the bladder's pillar.

DIGESTIVE SYSTEM INJURY

Injury to a digestive organ–small intestine, sigmoid colon, or rectum– can happen during any vaginal surgery that is hampered by adhesions. It is important to identify the lesion, because a satisfactory result is nearly always achievable by intraoperative treatment via a vaginal approach. Following any action of adhesiolysis one will, therefore, direct one's attention to the state of the digestive tract. Diagnosis of recto-sigmoidal injury can be facilitated by anal injection of a colorant.

A simple deperitonisation or sero-muscular lesion without opening of an organ is treated by a serous or sero-muscular suture using a resorbable thread.

An injury of the small intestine that is limited and neatly cut is closed by a transversal suture (extra-mucous, resorbable thread, separated stitches or overcast suture). In the case of a contused or enlarged lesion, or of a mesenteric haematoma, it is advisable to perform a limited segmental resection followed by anastomosis of the healthy tissue (haemostasis of the mesenteric triangle corresponding to the loop that is to be removed

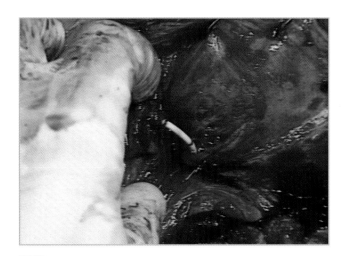

29.6 Repair of the injury shown in figure 29.5: the ureter has been supported by a probe.

as far as the mesenterium, clamping, sectioning, anastomosis in an extra-mucous plane using a resorbable thread (either by separated stitches or two semi-overcast sutures), verification of the tightness and vitality of the anastomosis).

An injury to the colon or rectum identified during the operation can generally be treated without colostomy, under the condition of satisfactory intestinal preparation. This justifies colic preparation by lavage for all procedures, using macromolecules for those operations carrying a high risk of a digestive injury (endometriosis, known major adhesions). The remaining abdominal cavity should in any case be immediately protected, the intestinal contents aspirated, the contaminated zones washed with Betadine-containing serum, and an antibiotic therapy administered for the intestinal flora. A simple neatly-cut colic or rectal injury can be treated by applying a tight suture in two planes. Drainage is not necessary. The procedure can be completed by anal dilatation.

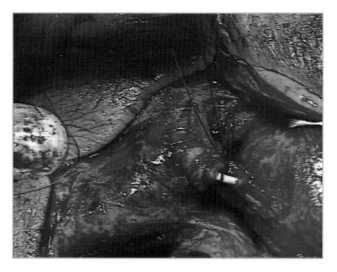

29.7 Extra-mucous suture of the ureter by four cardinal points using a single-strand, slow resorption thread.

CHAPTER 30

Intra- and postoperative haemorrhage

Guide to the reader

In this respect, vaginal surgery does not differ from any other approach: one must never loose one's calm, nor position forceps by chance, nor blindly insert the needle. One must blot, aspirate, identify the cause, and then treat it selectively.

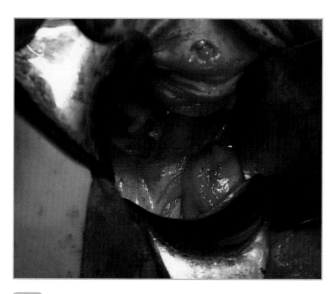

30.1 Posterior angle: the usual position for venous bleeding.
Here, it is clearly visible after a Wilkins (or Schauta) operation,
due to a detachment of the pelvic cellular tissue.

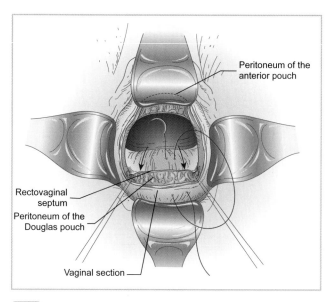

Peritoneum of the
anterior pouch

Rectovaginal
septum

Peritoneum of the
Douglas pouch

Vaginal section

30.2 Curative or preventive haemostasis of the posterior angle.
The "posterior angles" are indicated by an arrow.
This is a schematic representation of the preceding picture,
showing the execution of a haemostatic "X" stitch.

INTRAOPERATIVE HAEMORRHAGE

Bleeding of the vaginal section is the first and last demonstration of haemorrhage during the course of the procedure. Even though it is disturbing and not very aesthetic it does not represent any danger and ceases with the vaginal suture. A haemostatic infiltration performed prior to the incision can prevent such bleeding during the incision stage; however, a study carried out years back indicated that such an infiltration reduces the vaginal wall's anti-infectious defences.

A release of the cardinal ligaments or uterosacral ligaments is of little importance. The minor consequences this entails are felt if the threads are accidentally cut or ripped out. Haemostasis can easily be restored by taking hold of the vaginal mass, the ligament in question and the adjacent peritoneum with an "X" stitch.

At the end of the intervention, one often observes bleeding in the "posterior angles" , i.e. in the region where vaginal section and cellular pelvic tissue are opposite each other within the cardinal ligaments' insertion (figure 30.1), independently of whether haemostasis of the cardinal ligaments had been correctly performed or not. A systematic or curative suturing of this zone, with a resorbable stitch taking hold of the vaginal section, the cellular tissue of the recto-vaginal septum, and the lateral Douglas' pouch, allows the blocking of the posterior uterovaginal veins. These stitches (one for each "angle") must take hold of the vagina's and adjacent tissue's total thickness, as well as of the postero-lateral peritoneum; under such conditions, all blood vessels of the cardinal ligament are certain to be blocked, having at our disposal supportive tissue (the vagina) and a "dressing" that efficiently occludes the blood vessels (the peritoneum) (figure 30.2).

Problems with the uterine arteries are rare. One must not place forceps randomly. It is advisable to aspirate the blood in order to identify and selectively grasp the opened extremity with a toothless arterial forceps, and to visually position a haemostatic forceps at a distance sufficient to permit the placement of a simple ligature or self-blocking clip (figure 30.3). A setting ligature might worsen the bleeding if it perforates an element of the pedicle.

Uterine venous bleeding is less unusual. Coming from the uterus, venous bleeding can be controlled with a temporary forceps or even ignored if the procedure is liable to end rapidly (it often stops when traction is applied to the uterus). Parietal bleeding, however, must be brought under control. Two methods can be applied to this end:

– a technique analogous to the method described for arterial bleeding; however, more difficulties are encountered here, due to venous retraction and the more diffuse nature of the bleeding;

– if the bleeding originates in the posterior vaginal angle, close to the section of the cardinal and uterosacral ligaments, the already described realisation of "X" stitches is preferable.

Bleeding of the utero-ovarian pedicle following conserving hysterectomy is controlled by clamping and ligature: this pedicle is always accessible. Bleeding of the ovarian pedicle following vaginal annexectomy requires a more delicate treatment. If the pedicle remains in good shape and does not retract, the treatment is easy: it can be clamped and ligatured twice, or an Endoloop can be applied (*figure 30.4*). If the pedicle is retracted, we advise the use of a laparoscopic or laparotomic approach.

POSTOPERATIVE HAEMORRHAGES

Vaginal haemorrhage

Strong vaginal bleeding can originate from the vaginal section or from the operative region. Bleeding of the vaginal section may even be in the form of a jet: gauze pads are often not very efficient in this case, so an "X" stitch can easily be placed if the point of bleeding can be observed with a speculum. Bleeding of the operational region can be treated with gauze pads if there are no haemodynamic repercussions. Failure to control the bleeding with the gauze pads or any other emergency situation requires a return to the operating table. The surgical inspection always begins by a vaginal examination with the help of retractors. A visibly open blood vessel is taken care of as soon as possible. Bleeding from the pelvic region of indeterminate origin indicates a reopening of the vaginal suture followed by verification of the pedicles. Recourse to laparotomy is rare.

Internal acute haemorrhage

Circulatory shock accompanied by extreme anaemia without external haemorrhage requires a return to the operation table. Although one could commence with a quick vaginal investigation, one will usually opt for a laparoscopy if the haemodynamic state permits, or, should this not be the case, for laparotomy. After having aspirated the haemaperitoneum, identified the blood vessel in question, and selectively established its haemostasis by coagulation or ligature, a waiting period is observed for security reasons, during which a number of supplementary small haemorrhagic foci are usually identified and controlled. One finishes by washing the peritoneum with warm serum, avoiding traumatic aspiration of the operative region.

Haematoma

The haematoma is revealed by an inexplainable anaemia, pain, moderate hyperthermia, signs of compression or by a late perineal or suprapubic ecchymosis. The diagnosis is clinical and echographic, and the treatment usually conservative: reassure and observe the patient; if necessary, prescribe anti-inflammatory agents containing steroids or not. Evacuation is useful in certain instances.

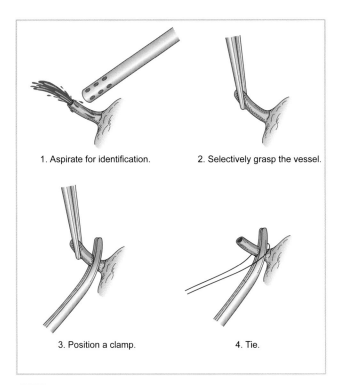

1. Aspirate for identification. 2. Selectively grasp the vessel.

3. Position a clamp. 4. Tie.

30.3 How to clamp and control a blood vessel.

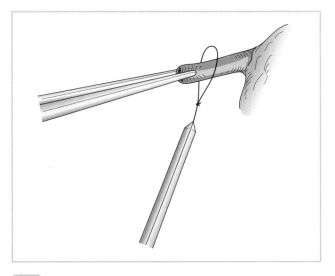

30.4 *Endoloop* onto a lombo-ovarian pedicle.
The pedicle has been grasped with a forceps positioned within the loop. One only needs to pull tight the knot of the loop.

Perspectives

This book describes the state-of-the-art of vaginal surgery, as it is practiced at the beginning of the 3rd millenium by three French surgeons that belong to three successive generations. The first of them (they are mentioned in order of age, which happens to correlate inversely with the efforts they put into this book's preparation!) started before the beginning of the "second French revolution", the revolution of endoscopic surgery. The second played a decisive part in this revolution and, more precisely, in its extension to oncological surgery by close collaboration with the former. The third belongs to the generation that can "chose its weapons" and who masters endoscopic surgery just as well as traditional surgery. The task of putting the whole story into perspective, to say where we came from, pinpoint the limits of present approaches and give a vision of the future, falls to the eldest.

HISTORY JUSTIFIES THE PRE-EMINENCE OF VAGINAL SURGERY

Vaginal surgery was born in an era when it was out of the question to operate otherwise than via a natural orifice. If the abdomen was opened, the patient was killed. By operating via the natural access routes, especially by extirpating the matrix and/or the ovaries through the vaginal route, one selected those patients that had enough courage to face the considerable risks the intervention brought along. Nevertheless, a good proportion of patients whose life was threatened by pelvic suppurations and/or cancers could be saved. Then, at the end of the 19th century, came the period where a series of developments rendered laparotomy possible, without sending the men and women that were so operated to certain death.

The decades around the turn of the 19th and 20th centuries saw the publication of a number of comparative studies. These concurrent necrologic reports were no reason for joy. Schauta, who operated cervix cancer patients via the natural access routes, saw a 10 % mortality. His student Wertheim, who operated via laparotomy, lost over 30 %. The numbers were terrible. The difference itself was all the more spectacular: the vaginal approach was three times less likely to result in death than abdominal surgery.

Then came the era when accelerating progress in intraoperative medicine meant that mortality on the operating table or in the days and weeks following the intervention became the exception. Abdominal surgery greatly profited from this, and, as a result, vaginal surgery became less used, since abdominal surgery was so much easier to learn and to perform. Once the mortality had radically declined, neither the surgeons nor the communities in which they were practicing could discern the differences. However, these differences persist, although it requires the power of statistical analyse performed on data collected across a whole continent to reveal them.

One of these studies was published in 1985 by the American epidemiologists Phillis Wingo and collaborators. It can be found in a journal in the database of the Commission of Professional and Hospital Activities. The data were collected during the years 1979 and 1980. Presumably, they represent 40 % of all hysterectomies performed in the United States of America during theses two years: 437,361 hysterectomies, 119,972 and 317, 389 of which were performed via a vaginal or abdominal approach, respectively. The numbers could be adjusted for age, race, and indication, separating those hysterectomies that were performed during the gravido-puerperal period or due to an invasive tumour. In all cases, mortality was higher if the patient was operated using an abdominal approach. If one excludes the hysterectomies carried out outside the gravido-puerperal period, as well as those performed due to an invasive cancer of the uterus or ovaries, i.e. restricting oneself to what seems to be solely attributable to the surgical intervention itself, the standardised totals are 6.9 and 2.3 per 1,000, respectively. At the beginning of the 20th century it was in the interest of the patient to be operated via a vaginal approach, and this has not changed at the beginning of the 21st century.

THE ROLE OF VAGINAL SURGERY IN TODAY'S GYNAECOLOGICAL SURGERY

Due to vaginal surgery's long, somewhat nostalgic, history, many young surgeons fear to appear backward if affirming a preference for this "timeless" access route. They are wrong. Vaginal surgery incorporates all criteria of modern surgery. The complications it brings along are less numerous and less important. What is more, the intraoperative stress appears to be significantly lower for those women for whom the after-effects are without complication. The patient suffers less, walks earlier, leaves the hospital earlier, has a shorter convalescence period, and forgets the difficult period she has been through much faster, which is in the end the most significant criterion of a successful surgical intervention. The complete absence of a visible scar obviously helps this process.

One can do everything, or nearly everything, via the vaginal route. This is a considerable advantage. The largest fibromas can be removed following the techniques described by French surgeons at the end of the 19th century, who have also coined the term "morcellation" that now belongs to the surgical vocabulary of all the world's languages. One can treat all adnexal diseases including cysts and endometrioses of the rectovaginal septum. One can even suspend prolapsed pelvic viscera to the pelvic wall via a vaginal approach... For nearly all abdominal operations there exists a vaginal alternative. But is this enough to exchange the whole classical repertoire for vaginal operations? Is it really necessary to follow the slogan "laparotomy = 0" in order to enter the "lion's club"? The answer is no. Surgeons are not paid to enter their name in the Guiness book of records, but to provide patients confiding themselves into their hands the most appropriate treatment. And there are some cases where the laparotomic access route is most advantageous. Furthermore, development of a new surgical approach, namely of laparoscopic surgery, over the last two decades profoundly changed the constellation. Today we have sufficient insight in order to discern the respective roles of the different access routes.

Treatment of diseases of uterine adnexa definitely do not belong within the scope of vaginal surgery. Pelvic infections and their sequels, ovarian and tubal tumours, extra-uterine pregnancies, as well as ovarian, peritoneal and retro-peritoneal endometrioses are treated via an abdominal approach: mostly via a laparoscopic access route, although laparotomy is still frequently applied, and one has to know when to favour one over the other. This is true for rectovaginal endometrioses that were shown to deeply and extensively invade the rectal wall and that must, therefore, be treated by an operative intervention that includes intestinal resection. In favourable cases, this surgery can be performed by combining vaginal and laparoscopic access routes. However, this intervention is often much more difficult than those for rectal cancers, where the most experienced experts discourage a systematic laparoscopic approach. In the majority of cases it is, therefore, advisable to operate using a laparotomic approach (combined or not with a vaginal approach).

Contrary to the situations we mentioned above, there are also those situations where the vaginal approach was believed not be acceptable, or only under laparoscopic assistance. At the end of the 1980s it was recommended to commence vaginal hysterectomy by laparoscopy in patients affected by risk factors rendering the former access route problematic. Since 1974 we have demonstrated that in 8 out of 10 cases, laparoscopy revealed that vaginal hysterectomy was absolutely possible in patients that would normally have been treated by laparotomy due to a preceding laparotomy. Operative laparoscopy allowed to go one step further and to section the adhesions if this was not done during the preceding laparotomy. It was rapidly discovered that such adhesions mostly concerned either the abdominal wall or the upper region of the internal genital organs and did not hamper, or only very weakly, the

realisation of vaginal hysterectomy. Consequently, we advise the surgeon to begin with vaginal hysterectomy, and continue with laparoscopy only in those cases where the problem cannot be treated via the initial access route. Complementary laparoscopy has now replaced preparatory laparoscopy. This concept is equally applied in cases where a bilateral annexectomy has been programmed, which does not represent an indication for a systematic laparoscopic preparation.

While the concept of vaginal hysterectomy with laparoscopic assistance is turning into an idea of the past, the concept of a purely laparoscopic hysterectomy is experiencing increasing success since the beginning of the 1990s. By preparing vaginal hysterectomy by laparoscopy, nothing, or not much, is won and precious time is lost. Performing the complete hysterectomy via laparoscopy is an altogether different scenario. The technique remained reserved to an elite during several years. The surgeons that had come up with the idea, namely the group around Maurice Bruhat in Clermont-Ferrand and especially Arnaud Wattiez, have managed to standardise the method so that it is now really reproducible. This technique's advantages are the same as those for vaginal hysterectomy: a surgery with minimal stress, a surgery that is easily forgotten. Even the disadvantage that was held against it at the beginning, namely occupying the operating table and surgical team for a longer time, is no longer true. We have personally experienced this by observing Arnaud Wattiez in cases where both access routes could be applied. The average operating times where exactly the same down to the minute. More recently, a prospective and randomised trial carried out by Mickaël Hohl in Baden (Switzerland) could even demonstrate that postoperative pains were reduced if hysterectomy was performed via laparoscopy. Is this the end of vaginal surgery?

VAGINAL SURGERY, SURGERY OF THE FUTURE

Vaginal surgery does not belong to the past. There are three good reasons why it has and will keep its place. The first is called technological development: this procedure profits from the same new technology that accelerate its rivals' progress. The second reason is at the conceptual level: vaginal surgery was the beginning of patient friendly surgery and its performance can still be enhanced, also in this domain. The third reason is at the cultural, and one can nearly say moral, level. Vaginal surgery is the surgery of gynaecologist-obstetricians and, in our times where doctors have justly to fulfil high

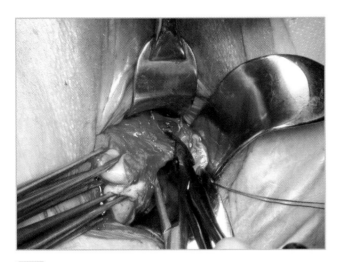

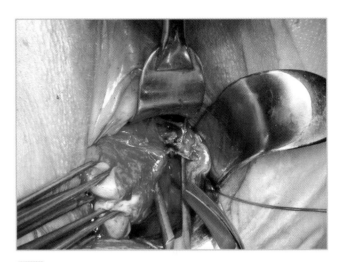

I.a Applying vascular sealing to treat the uterine artery during the course of vaginal hysterectomy.
The afferent branch of the uterine artery's loop has been dissected – it is tightly held in the clamp.

I.c Having been sealed, the artery is cut – note it's leathery aspect – note also, that the impaired tissue is restricted to the segment that was held in the forceps.

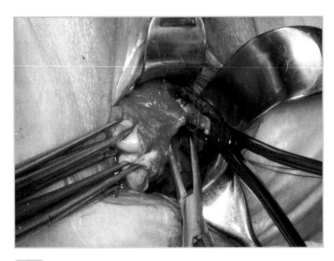

I.b The sealing is completed (it has been established by the microprocessors that are incorporated in the energy distribution circuit and the surgeon is informed of this via an acoustic signal).

demands, it is up to them to direct the operative interventions on the feminine genital organs.

Technological progress

It has been demonstrated that laparoscopic hysterectomy is superior to vaginal surgery, although this is not necessarily a direct result of the access route used. One can justly ask oneself whether the results obtained by Mickaël Hohl in his prospective and randomised trial were not due to the systematic and exclusive application of bipolar electro-coagulation of the blood vessels before cutting them, rather than due to the laparoscopic approach. This instrument helps to save time: "coagulating

and cutting" is done more rapidly than "clamping, cutting and ligaturing" or "stitching, ligaturing and cutting". The traumatic attrition of the stumps that are left in place is also less extensive. The inflammatory reaction and post-operative pains are reduced. If there were a technology that allowed the same to be done via a vaginal approach, the same results could be achieved via this access route. In fact, such a technology does exist. It is now possible to coagulate blood vessels such as the uterine blood vessels and their branches without having to dissect them first as is done during laparoscopic hysterectomy (endoscopic magnification renders this possible, but it is rather time-consuming: it partly uses up the time that is saved by not performing the ligatures).

The new technique is called "vascular sealing". Thanks to microprocessors that are incorporated in the circuitry providing electric energy to the tissues, the energy can be modulated according to the impedance of the tissue that is being treated. These tissues are held in a clamp, thus assuring and maintaining an appropriate pressure. The distributed current is pulsed, reaching 4 amperes at the height of each impulse. These physical properties of the current result in the biological effect that is best described as "vascular sealing": Once the distribution of energy is stopped by the microprocessors that have determined that the tissue's impedance has dropped to zero, the tissues in question have a leathery aspect, due to a fusion of the vascular walls that have been sealed one against the other (figure 1): one can now cut.

The clamps used during open surgery can equally be used for vaginal surgery. They are not very ergonomic (a bit too large, not bent enough), but the first trials of vaginal hysterectomy "without ligature" are very conclusive. Thanks to the vascular sealing instruments, vaginal hysterectomy can be performed in a shorter time-span and the aftermath appears to be much less painful (to the point where one of its fawning practitioners speaks of a hysterectomy "without pain"). Of course, one must be aware that, even though the new technology appears to be simple, the rules for anatomical surgery must in any case be known and respected: the surgical spaces have to be opened correctly and the structures separating them exposed accordingly so that the tissue can be sealing without risk. It is also important to note that vaginal surgery's rival techniques also benefit from the novel technologies: e.g. there exists a vascular sealing forceps, which carries a scalpel that can be advanced on command once tissue sealing has been achieved, confirmed by an acoustic signal. However, this instrument that saves a lot of time is rather voluminous and, since there is no curbed version, can only be comfortably used for laparotomic surgery. In summary, vaginal surgery still has its place and, without wanting to appear prophetic, one can bet that, with equal technological status, it will always remain the most advantageous approach for those indications where it can be applied.

The new concepts

Conceptual progress and technological progress are inseparable. Surgery for problems of pelvic stasis is a good example. At a conceptual level, it is nearly shocking to perform such an intervention with tissue whose impairment is known to be the origin of the pathology in question: at some point it is not possible to make new out of old. Since it is not possible to restore the initial qualities in impaired tissue, this has to be replaced or at least reinforced by using tissue that fulfil the requirements imposed by the natural equilibrium. Today, industry provides us with polypropylene, which exhibits next to ideal conditions. This synthetic material has the necessary resistance and elasticity, and it appears to be well tolerated, regardless whether inserted via the abdominal, laparotomic or laparoscopic access route. Now, surgeons also start to use it via a vaginal approach, and the first results are encouraging. The number of follow-up operations for the enclosure or ablation of prosthesis that are more or less "exposed" in the vaginal cavity is acceptable. However, this number is not zero either, which is reflected by the range of new products that are proposed monthly by producers and vendors.

With the working hypothesis that an ideal prosthesis does exist, it is certainly more logical to place it using a vaginal rather than an abdominal approach. The vesical base and/or ventral side of the rectum, the ptosis of which causes or accompanies the anterior and posterior colpoceles, can be exposed more easily and more completely using a vaginal approach. The prosthesis that will be placed in front of viscera in order to replace or strengthen the vesicovaginal and/or rectovaginal septum will better dress the ptosed organ. There is an open

competition as to how to cut and fix (or not to fix) the prostheses, which battle for the famous Lépine competition, awarded to the inventors of the can opener and other household gadgets, rather than for the Nobel prize. A non-exhaustive list of objects that are in vogue is given in chapter 23 of this book, to which I would now like to add the "Dirndl gauze" that I use for the treatment of larger cystoceles accompanied by a paravaginal dehiscence.

The Dirndl is the folkloric apron that Tyrolean barmaids wear in operettas. It is a truncated triangular or trapezoidal piece of tissue. The distance between the corners of the prosthesis' base amounts to 12 cm. The distance between the upper two corners is 4 cm. They are elongated by two straps (figure 2). The apron's 4 corners are designed to be fixed to the extremities of the arcus tendinous where the pelvic aponeurosis inserts itself, since we believe that the prosthesis should be fixed, without being stretched, at those points where the fascia that is to be replaced or strengthened inserts itself; is can thus perform its role as a security belt. The prosthesis' corners located at its base are attached by direct sutures performed directly in front of the ischial spine (cf. chapter 23). The prosthesis' upper corners should be fixed to the posterior side of the pubis. This procedure is easily executed via an abdominal approach, but very difficult to perform via a vaginal approach. Using the same artifice exploited for the positioning of sub-urethral slings via the trans-obturatory access route during urinary incontinence treatment (cf. chapter 24), the straps are pulled in order to precisely position the upper corners (near the upper inside corners of the obturated foramens).

The surgical aggressiveness can be further reduced by replacing the large median colpotomy that precedes opening of the paravesical spaces by two small transversal colpotomies, the lower of which is carried out at the vaginal insertion onto the uterine cervix while the uppermost is done at the junction of the median and lower thirds. The bladder's base is then separated from the vaginal wall's posterior side by a blunt dissection performed blindly between the two vaginal incisions. The plane that is thus created is enlarged in the front and back by lateral tunnels where the needle will pass through to pull on the four straps of the central prosthesis (this technique, thought up by Georges Eglin, requires the use of a prosthesis whose basis and top are both prolonged with straps). The anterior straps are guided just like the two extremities of the TVT strip. The posterior straps are guided either via a trans-obturatory approach (cf. chapter 22), or via a trans-perineal approach as described for the IVS' posterior straps (cf. chapter 23). The goal of this reduced aggressiveness is to limit the risk of exposure and rejection of the synthetic tissue. Until proof of the contrary, we prefer to proceed with a longitudinal median colpotomy, mobilise the bladder's base inside the "anatomical" vesicovaginal space, put the prosthesis into place and cleave the two lateral flaps in order to separate Halban's fascia, which will be used to perform a culdoplasty that will isolate the prosthesis from the vaginal suture. It is obvious that the winner of the Lépine competition's first prize is not yet decided... and vaginal surgery is all but dead.

The future of gynaecological surgery. The role of vaginal surgery... and of gynaecologist-obstetricians

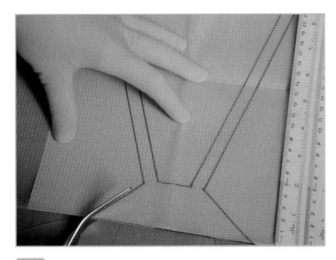

2.a The "Dirndl gauze" applied for the treatment of large cystocoeles with lateral vaginal desinsertion.
Cutting out the prosthesis: it resembles the apron worn by Tyrolean innkeepers (the Dirndl).

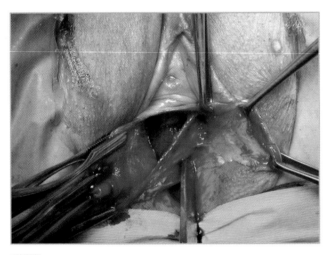

2.b The lower extremities of the trapezoid prosthesis have been fixed to the pelvic wall, just in front of the ischial spines (i.e. close to the posterior extremities of the tendinous arches), while the upper extremities have been pulled close to the supero-internal corners of the obturator hole via a trans-obturatory approach (i.e. close to the anterior extremities of the tendinous arches). The two vaginal flaps have been cleaved and will be superimposed onto the prosthesis, separating it from the vaginal suture.

Vaginal surgery is a surgery for gynaecologist-obstetricians. A general surgeon, especially if he is familiar with pelvic surgery, can just as well perform gynaecological operations... "with opened abdomen". Surgeons used to laparoscopic surgery will have no problem in performing even more advanced gynaecological interventions. However, both of them will be less at ease in regard to operations via natural access routes: it will not be their first choice. The gynaecologist-obstetrician, on the other hand, the surgeon that commenced his training in a delivery room and has assisted many others during childbirth, which are still performed via the natural access routes (provided that it lasts!), finds himself in his natural surroundings. However, the gynaecologist-obstetrician is not merely the one who is pushed most naturally towards the use of vaginal surgery. He his also in the best position to generally understand gynaecological surgery.

Radical trachelectomy, a technically elaborate technique, is an emblematic example for this. It is a complex, but above all demanding, intervention. Although it is based on rather simple principles, it requires a profound knowledge of the "vaginalist" surgical anatomy. This knowledge cannot be learned from textbooks. It requires experience to be acquired early and to be regularly refreshed at the operating table. Radical trachelectomy can be performed via laparotomy (this intervention was developed in 1932 by Aburel, who performed it via laparotomy). It can even be carried out via laparoscopy. Nevertheless, there exists a "quasi" universal consensus that the vaginal approach provides the best results. However, there is no way to achieve good results if one does not have a regular experience of Watkins' (or Schauta) operation. After all, radical trachelectomy is but a variant thereof (infra-fundal Watkin's intervention) and it is generally performed under difficult conditions, since the majority of candidates have never given birth and, therefore, have narrow genital routes.

The other aspect of radical trachelectomy concerns its gynaeco-obstetric consequences and the possibilities of preventing genital prolapses on the one hand, and cervico-isthmic incontinences on the other hand. By cutting the paracervical ligaments, the uterus is detached. In order to avoid a prolapse, which could in the long run result from such a disconnection, the Douglas' pouch, while suturing it, is purse-string stiched onto the posterior side of the isthmus, and the stumps of the paracervial ligaments firmly grasped, during a circular movement performed while taking up the peritoneal serosa. Before realising this "isthmo-suspension", one must have installed a cerclage around the uterine isthmus, using a non-resorbable thread that is usually used for preventive surrounding of the cervico-isthmic opening. This cerclage is positioned a little higher than the isthmorraphy point. Figure 3 illustrates the anatomical result as visualised during the final laparoscopic check-up: the cerclage is installed above the isthmus and the paracervical ligaments are reattached (especially the uterosacral ligaments). The gynaecologist-obstetrician's role does not end here. He has to treat eventual infertility linked to the poor quality of the cervical mucus, as well as the risks encountered during pregnancy due to the short size of the remaining uterine cervix.

In summary, radical trachelectomy is an affair for the gynaecologist-obstetrician. This operation nicely sums up the questions asked within the profession. The surgical indication and realisation of radical trachelectomy belong to the gynaecological cancerologist. Treatment of infertilities (IAC, FIV) is the field of specialists of the medical assistance for procreation, while post-intervention pregnancies should be surveyed by "level 3" maternal care units. Today, there are at least three other professions, parallel to that of gynaecologist-obstetrician: reproduction specialist, specialist of materno-fetal medicine, and gynaecological cancerologist. It is important that those carrying out one or another of these professions have originally undergone the same training, including both obstetrical and surgical practices. There should be no obstetricians that cannot operate, just as there is no use for gynaecological surgeons that have not commenced their training in a delivery room. This is not corporatist pleading. It is in the patients' interest to be treated by true specialists. One condition for these specialists, the gynaecologist-obstetricians, to retain the upper hand in their profession is that the techniques for vaginal surgery, which are not the only solutions, but which must still be considered as the first-choice treatments, continue to be developed and taught.

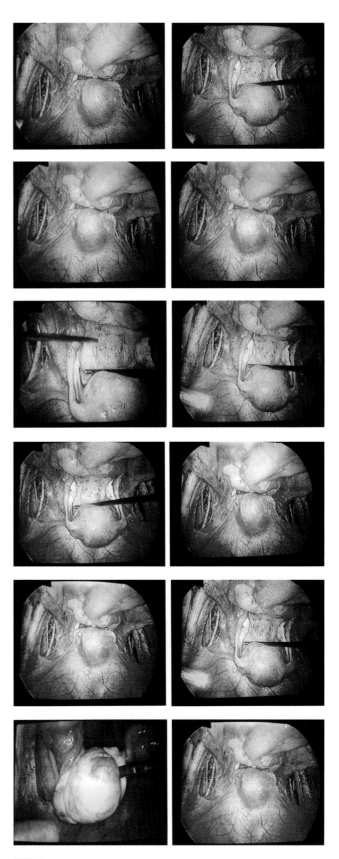

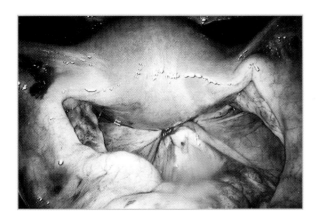

3.a Isthmic cerclage and reinsertion of the paracervical ligaments in the uterine isthmus' posterior side following radical trachelectomy.
Immediate endoscopic appearance.

3.b Endoscopic appearance after 6 months – note the absence of peritoneal adhesions and the new serosa covering the lateral spaces that have not been closed.

Index

Masson Éditeur
21, rue Camille Desmoulins
92789 Issy-Les-Moulineaux Cedex 9
Dépôt légal : novembre 2005

Achevé d'imprimer
par IME
25112 Baume-Les-Dames

Imprimé en France